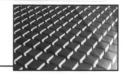

OBSESSIVE-COMPULSIVE
PERSONALITY DISORDER

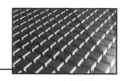

OBSESSIVE-COMPULSIVE PERSONALITY DISORDER

Edited by

Jon E. Grant, M.D., M.P.H., J.D.
Anthony Pinto, Ph.D.
Samuel R. Chamberlain, M.B.B.Chir., Ph.D., M.R.C.Psych.

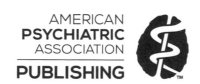

AMERICAN
PSYCHIATRIC
ASSOCIATION
PUBLISHING

Note: The authors have worked to ensure that all information in this book is accurate at the time of publication and consistent with general psychiatric and medical standards, and that information concerning drug dosages, schedules, and routes of administration is accurate at the time of publication and consistent with standards set by the U.S. Food and Drug Administration and the general medical community. As medical research and practice continue to advance, however, therapeutic standards may change. Moreover, specific situations may require a specific therapeutic response not included in this book. For these reasons and because human and mechanical errors sometimes occur, we recommend that readers follow the advice of physicians directly involved in their care or the care of a member of their family.

All names used in case vignettes are pseudonyms, and some details have been altered for privacy.

Books published by American Psychiatric Association Publishing represent the findings, conclusions, and views of the individual authors and do not necessarily represent the policies and opinions of American Psychiatric Association Publishing or the American Psychiatric Association.

If you wish to buy 50 or more copies of the same title, please go to www.appi.org/special discounts for more information.

Copyright © 2020 American Psychiatric Association Publishing
ALL RIGHTS RESERVED
First Edition
Manufactured in the United States of America on acid-free paper
23 22 21 20 19   5 4 3 2 1
American Psychiatric Association Publishing
800 Maine Avenue SW
Suite 900
Washington, DC 20024-2812
www.appi.org

Library of Congress Cataloging-in-Publication Data
Names: Grant, Jon E., editor. | Pinto, Anthony, editor. | Chamberlain, Samuel, editor. | American Psychiatric Association Publishing, issuing body.
Title: Obsessive-compulsive personality disorder / edited by Jon E. Grant, Anthony Pinto, Samuel R. Chamberlain.
Description: Washington, D.C. : American Psychiatric Association Publishing, [2020] | Includes bibliographical references and index. |
Identifiers: LCCN 2019034531 (print) | LCCN 2019034532 (ebook) | ISBN 9781615372249 (paperback) | ISBN 9781615372805 (ebook)
Subjects: MESH: Obsessive-Compulsive Disorder—therapy | Obsessive-Compulsive Disorder—diagnosis | Compulsive Personality Disorder—therapy | Compulsive Personality Disorder—diagnosis
Classification: LCC RC533 (print) | LCC RC533 (ebook) | NLM WM 176 | DDC 616.85/227–dc23
LC record available at https://lccn.loc.gov/2019034531
LC ebook record available at https://lccn.loc.gov/2019034532
British Library Cataloguing in Publication Data
A CIP record is available from the British Library.

Contents

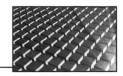

CONTRIBUTORS

Lucy Albertella, Ph.D.
Research Fellow, Brain and Mental Health Laboratory, Monash Institute of Cognitive and Clinical Neurosciences and School of Psychological Sciences, Monash University, Clayton, Victoria, Australia

Bekir B. Artukoglu, M.D.
Postdoctoral fellow, Yale Child Study Center, New Haven, Connecticut

Michael H. Bloch, M.D., M.S.
Associate Professor, Yale Child Study Center, New Haven, Connecticut

Julius Burkauskas, Ph.D.
Clinical Psychologist, Laboratory of Behavioral Medicine, Neuroscience Institute, Lithuanian University of Health Sciences, Palanga, Lithuania

Samuel R. Chamberlain, M.B./B.Chir., Ph.D., M.R.C.Psych.
Psychiatrist and Clinical Fellow, Department of Psychiatry, University of Cambridge; Cambridge and Peterborough NHS Foundation Trust, Cambridge, UK

Emil F. Coccaro, M.D.
Clinical Neuroscience Research Unit, Department of Psychiatry and Behavioral Neuroscience, Pritzker School of Medicine, University of Chicago, Chicago, Illinois

Scott J. Crow, M.D.
Professor of Psychiatry, University of Minnesota, Minneapolis, Minnesota

D. Ashkawn Ehsan, M.D.
Assistant Professor, Department of Psychiatry and Behavioral Neuroscience, University of Chicago, Chicago, Illinois

Naomi A. Fineberg, M.B.B.S., M.A., M.R.C.Psych.
Professor of Psychiatry, University of Hertfordshire, Hatfield, UK; Consultant Psychiatrist, Highly Specialized Obsessive Compulsive Disorder and Body Dysmorphic Disorder Service, Hertfordshire Partnership University NHS Foundation Trust, Welwyn Garden City, UK

Leonardo F. Fontenelle, M.D., Ph.D.
Professor, Monash Institute of Cognitive and Clinical Neurosciences, Monash University, Clayton, Victoria, Australia

Jon E. Grant, M.D., M.P.H., J.D.
Professor, Department of Psychiatry, University of Chicago, Chicago, Illinois

Y.C. Janardhan Reddy, M.D.
Professor of Psychiatry and Head, Obsessive-Compulsive Disorder (OCD) Clinic, Department of Psychiatry, National Institute of Mental Health and Neurosciences (NIMHANS), Bangalore, India

Angeli Landeros-Weisenberger, M.D.
Associate Research Scientist, Yale Child Study Center, New Haven, Connecticut

Christine Lochner, M.D.
Department of Psychiatry, Stellenbosch University, Cape Town, South Africa

Anthony Pinto, Ph.D.
Associate Professor of Psychiatry, Donald and Barbara Zucker School of Medicine at Hofstra/Northwell, The Zucker Hillside Hospital; Director, Northwell Health OCD Center, Glen Oaks, New York

Julliana N. Quintas, M.D.
Psychiatrist and mastership candidate, Obsessive, Compulsive, and Anxiety Spectrum Research Program, Institute of Psychiatry, Federal University of Rio de Janeiro, Rio de Janeiro, Brazil

Dan J. Stein, M.D.
Department of Psychiatry and Mental Health, University of Cape Town, Cape Town, South Africa

Michael G. Wheaton, Ph.D.
Assistant Professor, Department of Psychology, Barnard College, New York

Kaitlyn Wright, B.A.
Graduate student, School of Social Work, University of Michigan, Ann Arbor, Michigan

DISCLOSURE OF INTERESTS

The following contributors to this book have indicated a financial interest in or other affiliation with a commercial supporter, a manufacturer of a commercial product, a provider of a commercial service, a nongovernmental organization, and/or a government agency, as listed below:

Michael H. Bloch, M.D., M.S. is on the Scientific Advisory Board of Therapix Biosciences and receives research support from Biohaven Pharmaceuticals, Neurocrine Biosciences, Janssen Pharmaceuticals, and Therapix Biosciences. He also receives research support from the National Institutes of Health, Tourette Association of America, Brain and Behavior Research Foundation (formerly National Alliance for Research on Schizophrenia and Depression [NARSAD]), and the Patterson Foundation.

Samuel R. Chamberlain, M.B./B.Chir., Ph.D., M.R.C.Psych. consults for Cambridge Cognition, Shire, P1Vital, Ieso Digital Health, and Promentis Pharmaceuticals. He receives a stipend for his role as associate editor at *Neuroscience and Biobehavioral Reviews* and at *Comprehensive Psychiatry*.

Jon E. Grant, M.D., M.P.H., J.D. has received research grants from National Institute of Mental Health, National Center for Responsible Gaming, and Forest and Roche Pharmaceuticals. He receives yearly compensation from Springer Publishing for acting as editor-in-chief of the *Journal of Gambling Studies* and has received royalties from Oxford University Press, American Psychiatric Association Publishing, Norton Press, and McGraw-Hill.

The following contributors have indicated that they have no financial interests or other affiliations that represent or could appear to represent a competing interest with the contributions to this book: **Bekir B. Artukoglu, M.D.; Angeli Laneros-Weisenberger, M.D.**

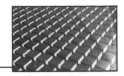

INTRODUCTION

Beginning in 2001, the National Epidemiologic Survey on Alcohol and Related Conditions (NESARC) was the first national survey in the United States to assess rates of the DSM-IV (and later DSM-5) personality disorders (American Psychiatric Association 1994, 2013). The NESARC data showed that obsessive-compulsive personality disorder (OCPD) not only was the most common personality disorder, with a prevalence of 7.8%, but also was approximately two times more common than any other personality disorder (Grant et al. 2004). Notably, however, a PubMed search for OCPD yields only about 300 publications, whereas a search for borderline personality disorder yields almost 8,000. Given the high prevalence of OCPD and the relative lack of research in this area, we felt that a textbook devoted exclusively to OCPD was needed to inform people of what is currently known about OCPD and to highlight important areas that need more investigation.

The study of OCPD is important from both clinical and research perspectives. OCPD not only is prevalent but also is associated with significant morbidity (lower quality of life and problems in overall psychosocial functioning) (Mancebo et al. 2005; Pinto et al. 2014) and increased health costs (Diedrich and Voderholzer 2015; Fineberg et al. 2014). Recent years have seen a rapid increase in understanding of the phenomenology, neurobiology, and psychology of this disorder, as well as of the domains of perfectionism, cognitive rigidity, and procrastination (all key domains underlying OCPD). Unfortunately, although many clinicians encounter patients with OCPD (elevated rates are observed in patients with a variety of mental health disorders), clinicians often do not diagnose OCPD, may incorrectly diagnose it as obsessive-compulsive disorder (OCD) or attention-deficit/hyperactivity disorder, and are frequently unaware of the treatment options for the disorder.

Many clinicians are also unaware of the personal consequences of OCPD. This lack of awareness in turn leads physicians and psychologists to ignore OCPD in both mental health and primary care settings. Toward that end, Chapter 1, "History and Epidemiology of OCPD," presents the evolution of OCPD in DSM and its place in the World Health Organization's *International Classification of Diseases* (ICD) nomenclature. A primary aim of this book is to educate treatment providers about OCPD. In furtherance of this aim, the text addresses the diagnosis and evaluation of individuals with OCPD. Many people can readily spot personality characteristics of themselves within the OCPD criteria; understanding when these characteristics rise to the level of a disorder is important. Chapter 2, "Diagnosis and Clinical Features of OCPD," addresses this issue and highlights phenomenologically how the disorder is different in degree, but not in kind, from the personality characteristics that many of us exhibit.

Clinicians' lack of awareness of OCPD often stems from the diagnostic confusion between OCPD and other mental health problems. Four chapters in this book focus on common mental health disorders that are often difficult to disentangle from OCPD. First, Chapter 3 takes on comparisons between OCPD and the two most common misdiagnoses, OCD and hoarding disorder. The chapter provides a thorough approach to differentiating these disorders, because they may require unique treatment interventions. OCPD has also been linked with eating disorders (discussed in Chapter 4), impulse-control disorders (Chapter 5), and aggression (Chapter 6), either as a co-occurring personality disorder to these other problems; as the primary problem with dysfunctional eating, impulsivity, and aggression as symptoms of the personality pathology; or as a compensatory reaction to these other issues.

A growing area of interest in mental health is how the presentation of psychiatric disorders may or may not be influenced by gender and/or cultural factors. This topic, discussed in Chapter 7, not only is of research interest but also may affect how treatment providers diagnose and assist people with OCPD based on culture and gender.

Treatment providers often assume that "one size fits all" in terms of treatment. This may not be the case for OCPD, which is a complex personality pathology with a potentially heterogeneous etiology. Much of the treatment literature on OCPD has been based on different theories regarding OCPD's similarities to other disorders (e.g., OCD) or on the primary domain that providers feel drives the personality pathology (e.g., perfectionism, cognitive rigidity). As a result, treatment providers caring for people with OCPD have multiple treatment options at their disposal. Chapter 9, on psychotherapeutic treatment approaches, distills the various cognitive-behavioral therapies for OCPD, the rationale behind their use, their effectiveness in helping people with OCPD, and the limitations of the current psychological interventions. Similarly, Chapter 10, on pharmacological treatment approaches, reviews the current state of drug treatment for OCPD and the rationale for what has been tried.

To further enhance treatment options, both treatment providers and researchers look to possible developmental, psychological, and behavioral etiologies, as well as the deeper neurobiological underpinnings of the disorder. Therefore, these realms of explanations for the disorder are examined in this book. Chapter 8, on psychobiology of OCPD, examines neurobiological systems that have been associated with OCPD or aspects of the disorder, and Chapter 11 ("Impact of Personality Disorders on Parenting") probes the complex interplay between parenting and OCPD. The neurobiological and psychological understanding of OCPD may be useful in developing new treatment approaches for this disabling disorder and may provide deeper understanding of a range of disorders or behaviors also driven by some of the core OCPD domains.

One complicating factor in the analysis of OCPD is that not everyone with this disorder thinks of it as a problem. In truth, many of the individual criteria, when examined in isolation, are often highly sought-after personality traits (e.g., excessive dedication to work). Therefore, Chapter 12 makes a distinction between obsessive-compulsive personality and OCPD and argues that aspects of obsessive-compulsive personality may have positive longitudinal associations across the lifespan, especially when viewed at the level of the general population—or in particular educational or work contexts—rather than in clinical cohorts. This view may suggest that instead of having a treatment goal of eliminating the disorder, interventions should seek to dial down the intensity of the various domains; it also suggests that future work should explore latent phenotypes of OCPD rather than only the categorical diagnosis as a unitary entity.

Another aim of this volume is to persuade readers that work on OCPD is extremely important. Each of the chapters addresses this theme in one way or another. Many of the chapters emphasize the dysfunction associated with OCPD. Although OCPD may not appear to represent a major public health problem at first blush, on closer examination it represents key elements of human existence taken to such an extreme level to result in personal or interpersonal suffering. Other chapters highlight the ways in which OCPD provides unique insight into other aspects of human behavior, such as rigidity belief systems, perfectionism, and striving to improve.

In summary, OCPD represents an important and yet remarkably largely neglected area of clinical care, especially given its high population prevalence. As the authors of the chapters in this volume eloquently attest, extraordinary progress has been made in understanding the clinical presentation and diagnosis of OCPD. Despite this progress, many treatment providers who encounter OCPD do not diagnose it and do not know how best to address it clinically. We hope that clinicians who desire to make more informed decisions regarding the well-being of those with OCPD will find this text valuable, as will researchers in OCPD and its allied fields.

Jon E. Grant, M.D., M.P.H., J.D.
Samuel R. Chamberlain, M.B.B.Chir., Ph.D., M.R.C.Psych.

REFERENCES

American Psychiatric Association: Diagnostic and Statistical Manual of Mental Disorders, 4th Edition. Washington, DC, American Psychiatric Association, 1994

American Psychiatric Association: Diagnostic and Statistical Manual of Mental Disorders, 5th Edition. Arlington, VA, American Psychiatric Association, 2013

Diedrich A, Voderholzer U: Obsessive-compulsive personality disorder: a current review. Curr Psychiatry Rep 17(2):2, 2015 25617042

Fineberg NA, Chamberlain SR, Goudriaan AE, et al: New developments in human neurocognition: clinical, genetic, and brain imaging correlates of impulsivity and compulsivity. CNS Spectr 19(1):69–89, 2014 24512640

Grant BF, Hasin DS, Stinson FS, et al: Prevalence, correlates, and disability of personality disorders in the United States: results from the National Epidemiologic Survey on Alcohol and Related Conditions. J Clin Psychiatry 65(7):948–958, 2004 15291684

Mancebo MC, Eisen JL, Grant JE, et al: Obsessive compulsive personality disorder and obsessive compulsive disorder: clinical characteristics, diagnostic difficulties, and treatment. Ann Clin Psychiatry 17(4):197–204, 2005 16402751

Pinto A, Steinglass JE, Greene AL, et al: Capacity to delay reward differentiates obsessive-compulsive disorder and obsessive-compulsive personality disorder. Biol Psychiatry 75(8):653–659, 2014 24199665

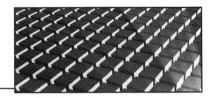

CHAPTER 1

HISTORY AND EPIDEMIOLOGY OF OCPD

Julius Burkauskas, Ph.D.
Naomi A. Fineberg, M.B.B.S., M.A., M.R.C.Psych.

Case Vignette

Andrew is a 45-year-old accountant. His wife has brought him for consultation because he is depressed. He is not sleeping or eating, has lost 11 pounds, and is anxious all the time about losing his job. He reports that he has recently been struggling at work since the firm was taken over by new employers who are expecting him to complete more auditing work in less time, and he is highly anxious about making mistakes. He says he has always been extremely conscientious and reports difficulties delegating his work as well as a tendency to get easily distracted by details. Andrew cites as an example the fact that he would find small discrepancies, such as pennies missing at audit, highly distracting and spends longer then he should searching for the source of insignificant error. As a result, he is slower than most of his colleagues, but he claims that the quality of his work is of the highest standard and that previously his meticulousness was not seen as a problem. He is angry and

1

critical of his new employers for taking a different attitude. He thinks he has been unfairly treated and is not prepared to change the way he works. He admits to long-standing workaholic tendencies, has almost no social life apart from his relationship with his wife, and holds judgmental attitudes. He hoards outdated electrical items in the shed. He is noted to make poor eye contact. His wife describes him as obstinate, rigid, and stubborn but also loyal and trustworthy.

Obsessive-compulsive personality disorder (OCPD) is characterized by a pervasive and maladaptive pattern of excessive perfectionism, preoccupation with orderliness and details, and need for control over one's environment (Wheaton and Pinto 2017). The *Diagnostic and Statistical Manual of Mental Disorders*, 5th Edition (DSM-5) defines *personality disorders* as impairments in personality (self and interpersonal) functioning and the presence of pathological personality traits and categorizes personality disorders into three different clusters (A, B, and C) based on descriptive similarities. OCPD is classified as one of three Cluster C ("anxious-fearful") personality disorder types. DSM-5 specifically emphasizes that OCPD traits of orderliness, perfectionism, and mental and interpersonal control are expressed at the expense of flexibility, openness, and efficiency (American Psychiatric Association 2013). Developers of the *International Classification of Diseases*, 11th Revision (ICD-11), are moving toward a dimensional model of personality disorder assessment, which involves an evaluation of both personality disorder severity—mild, moderate, or severe—and the presence of five stylistic trait domains—negative affectivity, detachment, disinhibition, dissociality, and anankastia (World Health Organization 2018). Notably, the DSM-5 definition of OCPD considerably overlaps with the ICD-11 proposed trait of *anankastia*, which is described as rigid perfectionism as well as controlling behavior and situations to ensure conformity to standards (World Health Organization 2018).

Despite the recent developments in diagnostic classification, OCPD remains a relatively underexplored area of psychiatry, and its nosological status remains controversial (Fineberg et al. 2015). In particular, OCPD's relationship to other DSM-5 obsessive-compulsive and related disorders (OCRDs), such as obsessive-compulsive disorder (OCD) and hoarding disorder, has been debated in the literature (Fineberg et al. 2007; Murphy et al. 2010; Pollak 1979, 1987). Although current research studies provide evidence that patients with OCRDs have higher rates of many personality disorders (not only OCPD) (Bulli et al. 2016; Pena-Garijo et al. 2013; Zhang et al. 2015), the answer to the question of whether OCPD represents a mental disorder that falls within or outside the OCRD family varies depending on the method of inquiry used (e.g., disordered personality traits, neurodevelopmental profiles, neuropsychological mechanisms) (Fineberg et al. 2007).

ORIGINS OF THE DIAGNOSIS

Over the past century, there have been major changes in the way OCPD is diagnosed, even though understanding of the diagnosis is still heavily influenced by psychoanalytic theory. Janet (1904) was among the first to propose criteria for personality features thought to be relevant for obsessions and compulsions. He described traits of perfectionism, indecisiveness, and reserved emotions as cardinal features for the development of *psychasthenic illness* (Pitman 1984). The illness Janet described now probably would be considered to be OCD. Sigmund Freud's work (Freud 1908) on obsessive personality or *anal-erotic character style*, which described such traits as orderliness, parsimony, obstinacy, and the need for control (Jones 1918), also contributed greatly to modern understanding of the diagnosis of OCPD.

Lewis (1936), however, suggested that anal-erotic character style traits are also commonly found among patients without obsessions. He described two types of obsessional personality: "the one obstinate, morose, irritable, the other vacillating, uncertain of himself, submissive" (p. 325).

Abraham's (1966) proposed definition of anal character included the concept of *perfectionism* as one of the core features. Abraham believed that traits of perfectionism might *help* an individual to be conscientious and persistent with work but at the same time could produce *negative affective states* resulting in maladaptive social and interpersonal consequences, such as difficulty working cooperatively. Many authors at that time thought that these character traits precede OCD development and exacerbate OCD symptoms (Kraepelin and Quen 1990; Pitman 1984).

DEFINITION OF OCPD IN DSM

DSM-I (American Psychiatric Association 1952) introduced *compulsive personality disorder*, defined by chronic, excessive, or obsessive concern and by adherence to standards of conscience or of conformity. A strong emphasis was placed on rigidity, reduced capacity for relaxation, over-inhibition, overconscientiousness, and an inordinate capacity for work.

In DSM-II (American Psychiatric Association 1968), the name of the condition was changed to *obsessive-compulsive personality disorder*, and individuals with this disorder were described as rigid, over-inhibited, over-conscientious, and over-dutiful. DSM-II also introduced the term *anankastic personality* to reduce confusion between the personality disorder and OCD. However, this new term was subsequently removed from following editions.

In DSM-III (American Psychiatric Association 1980), the name was changed back to *compulsive personality disorder*, and a feature of "restricted ability to express warm and tender emotions" was included, which once again distinguished the personality disorder from OCD. This new feature closely resembled what we would consider, in modern classification, to be traits of autistic spectrum disorders. Indeed, OCPD and autistic spectrum disorders are commonly mistaken for each other, at least in the clinical psychiatry setting (Gadelkarim et al., in press).

Additional personality features included in the DSM-III definition were perfectionism, insistence that others submit to the individual's way of doing things, excessive devotion to work and productivity, and indecisiveness (American Psychiatric Association 1980). DSM-III-R (American Psychiatric Association 1987) included new criteria, including preoccupation with details (to the extent that the major point of the activity is lost), scrupulousness, inflexibility, lack of generosity, and hoarding. Presence of five criteria were required for the diagnosis.k

The eight current DSM-5 criteria for OCPD diagnosis have not changed substantially since DSM-IV was introduced in 1994 (American Psychiatric Association 1994). Those criteria are 1) preoccupation with details, 2) perfectionism interfering with task completion, 3) excessive devotion to work and productivity, 4) overconscientiousness, 5) hoarding, 6) reluctance to delegate, 7) miserly spending style, and 8) rigidity and stubbornness. The same criteria for diagnosing OCPD were used in DSM-IV-TR (American Psychiatric Association 2000) and DSM-5 (American Psychiatric Association 2013). The OCPD diagnosis requires that at least four (or more) of the listed specific criteria be met. Current diagnostic criteria for OCPD allow different combinations of symptoms that could lead to a diagnosis, showing possible complexity and symptom variation of the same disorder. However, the change from five criteria (in DSM-III-R) to four criteria (in DSM-IV and DSM-5) has arguably lowered the diagnostic threshold. Of the DSM-5 criteria, hoarding is perhaps the least specific for OCPD, in that it also appears in the description of OCD and counts as the principal criterion for the new diagnosis of hoarding disorder (an OCRD). Indeed, suggestions have been made that in the future OCPD may be more appropriately classified within the OCRDs, owing to the growing recognition of overlapping clinical and biological factors (Stein et al. 2016).

PREVALENCE

According to DSM-5, OCPD is one of the most common personality disorders in the general population, with a prevalence ranging from 2.1% to 7.9% (American Psychiatric Association 2013, p. 681). Although DSM-5 reports that men are twice as likely as women to be diagnosed with OCPD, data to support this finding are limited and under investigation (Carter et al. 1999; Grant et al. 2012; Maier et al. 1992; Nestadt et al. 1991; Torgersen et al. 2001).

OCPD is also one of the most commonly identified personality disorders in clinical samples, in both psychiatric outpatient (Stuart et al. 1998; Zimmerman et al. 2005) and inpatient (Rossi et al. 2000) settings. The prevalence is reported to increase to around 25% in clinical psychiatry samples (Ansell et al. 2010; Pena-Garijo et al. 2013) and to more than 30% in OCD services (Garyfallos et al. 2010; Starcevic et al. 2013).

It is worth noting that prevalence of OCPD in community populations may differ according to the diagnostic manual and questionnaire used. When OCPD was assessed using DSM-III-R criteria, prevalence rates ranged from approximately 1% (Moldin et al. 1994) to 5% (Bodlund et al. 1993), with a median prevalence of 2.2%. For example, in a large Australian community study ($N=10,641$) using DSM-III, findings suggested an OCPD prevalence of 3% (Jackson and Burgess 2000). However, when DSM-IV criteria were used in studies in the United States (Samuels et al. 2002) and Turkey (Dereboy et al. 2014), prevalence of OCPD ranged more widely from 1% up to 14% (Dereboy et al. 2014; Samuels et al. 2002), with a median prevalence of 4.6%. One of the largest U.S. community studies to date ($N=43,093$) estimated the OCPD prevalence at 8% using DSM-IV criteria (Grant et al. 2004, 2012). The discrepancy could be explained by the change in diagnostic algorithms from DSM-III to the more permissive DSM-IV. However, because no studies have directly compared prevalence rates for the different nosological sets of OCPD as described in DSM-III and DSM-IV, the definitive reason for the discrepancy has yet to be determined.

Furthermore, the prevalence of OCPD as reported in the DSM-5 review differs considerably from that reported in the DSM-IV review, despite the fact that the diagnostic criteria have barely changed. This variation may be partly explained by the fact that the DSM-5 committee had access to a greater number of community studies, which had been performed since the preparation of the previous edition.

Volkert et al. (2018) provided the most up-to-date systematic review and meta-analysis of the prevalence of personality disorders in the general adult population in Western countries (five studies with 55,216 individuals). They reported an overall OCPD prevalence rate of 2.36% (95% confidence interval [CI], 1.50%–3.39%). They also found considerable heterogeneity in the prevalence of OCPD, which they attributed to the increased risk of bias associated with the use of self-rated rather than expert-rated diagnostic assessments. Research has concluded that studies using the self-rating assessments of the Personality Diagnostic Questionnaire (PDQ) and Structured Clinical Interview for DSM-IV Axis II Personality Disorders (SCID-II) consistently report higher prevalence rates for the majority of personality disorders in general. A discrepancy also was reported for OCPD specifically: the prevalence estimate reported for self-rated diagnostic assessment was significantly higher than that reported for expert-rated assessments (4.32% vs. 2.36%) (Volkert et al. 2018). One possible explanation could be that some of the self-rated traits of OCPD, such as perfectionism or extreme responsibility, might actually be desirable in Western cultures and associated more with general orientation toward achievement. Thus, respondents might choose to fill the questionnaire in a socially desirable form.

SYSTEMATIC PREVALENCE ANALYSIS

For the purposes of this chapter, we used a systematic approach to identify studies to include in an updated prevalence report. We searched English language databases (Medline, PsycInfo) from 1980 to 2018 for studies reporting OCPD prevalence in otherwise healthy community samples. Studies were included if they 1) reported prevalence rates of OCPD in the community sample or general adult population (minimum mean age 18 years), 2) identified OCPD with standardized diagnostics according to DSM-III to DSM-5 or ICD-10, and 3) were published in English or had an English abstract with reported prevalence. Further details of the search technique are available from the authors. The search produced 27 articles reporting 26 studies involving more than 78,00 participants suitable for prevalence analysis (Table 1–1).

This analysis included a greater number of studies than did the meta-analysis by Volkert et al. (2018) mainly because of the addition of studies published in 2017 and 2018 (Gawda and Czubak 2017; Irfan et al. 2018). As expected, the observed prevalence differed between studies using DSM-III/DSM-III-R and those using DSM-IV. The studies using DSM-III/DSM-III-R reported considerably lower prevalence rates (2.8% [95% CI, 1.8%–4.1%]), on average by 3 percentage points, than studies using DSM-IV (5.8% [95% CI, 3.2%–9.2%]). Studies using self-rated OCPD diagnoses also produced higher reported prevalence rates than studies using observer-rated scales. For example, two studies employing self-rated scales reported unusually high OCPD prevalence rates (Becoña et al. 2013; Dereboy et al. 2014), ranging from 14.1% up to 36.6%. Researchers' preference for using self-rated methods for OCPD assessment may be because of the time and expense required to administer clinical interviews. In general, we found that there is still a shortage of adequate population-based studies with sufficient sample sizes to accurately determine the prevalence of OCPD. Also, none of the studies so far have used DSM-5 criteria to estimate the prevalence of OCPD. A cross-national database of OCPD epidemiology in the general adult population would allow better assessment of the worldwide prevalence of the disorder.

TABLE 1–1. Prevalence of obsessive-compulsive personality disorder (OCPD) according to DSM-III/DSM-III-R and DSM-IV criteria

Authors	Country[a]	Population	Rating[b]	Number of subjects	Instrument of evaluation[c]	Version	OCPD prevalence range
Reich et al. 1989	US	Community sample of adults	SR	235	PDQ	DSM-III	10.6–20.1
Zimmerman and Coryell 1989	US	First-degree relatives of normal controls	OR	797	SIDP	DSM-III	1.2–3.2
Maier et al. 1992	DE	Control probands recruited in the general population	OR	452	SCID-II	DSM-III-R	1.1–4.0
Black et al. 1993	US	Comparison subjects recruited through advertisement	OR	127	SIDP	DSM-III	3.8–14.0
Bodlund et al. 1993	SE	Students and their partners	SR	133	SCID-Screen	DSM-III-R	1.7–9.6
Samuels et al. 1994	US	Community sample of adults	OR	762	SPE	DSM-III	0.5–2.2
Moldin et al. 1994	US	General population	OR	302	PDE	DSM-III-R	0.1–2.4
Klein et al. 1995	US	Normal control subjects and their relatives	OR	229	PDE	DSM-III-R	1.0–5.6
Lenzenweger et al. 1997	US	Students	OR	258	IPDE	DSM-III-R	0–1.4

TABLE 1–1. Prevalence of obsessive-compulsive personality disorder (OCPD) according to DSM-III/DSM-III-R and DSM-IV criteria (*continued*)

Authors	Country[a]	Population	Rating[b]	Number of subjects	Instrument of evaluation[c]	Version	OCPD prevalence range
Jackson and Burgess 2000	AU	Community sample of adults	SR and OR	10,641	IPDE	DSM-III	2.8–3.4
Torgersen et al. 2001	NO	Community sample of adults	OR	2,053	SIDP-R	DSM-III-R	1.4–2.6
Ekselius et al. 2001	SE	Community sample of adults	SR	557	DIP-Q	DSM-IV	5.6–10.3
Samuels et al. 2002	US	Community sample of adults	OR	742	IPDE	DSM-IV	0.6–2.3
Albert et al. 2004	IT	Subjects invited through family doctor	OR	101	SCID-II	DSM-IV	0.6–8.4
Crawford et al. 2005	US	Community sample of young adults	OR	716	SCID-II	DSM-IV	3.3–6.6
Coid et al. 2006	UK	Community sample of adults	OR	626	SCID-II	DSM-IV	1.0–3.3
Moran et al. 2006	AU	Community sample of adults	OR	1,943	SAP	DSM-IV	4.8–7.0
Wu et al. 2006	US	Students	SR	418	SNAP-2	DSM-IV	2.8–7.0
Lindal and Stefansson 2009	IS	Community sample of adults	SR	805	DIP-Q	DSM-IV	5.6–9.4

TABLE 1–1. Prevalence of obsessive-compulsive personality disorder (OCPD) according to DSM-III/DSM-III-R and DSM-IV criteria *(continued)*

Authors	Country[a]	Population	Rating[b]	Number of subjects	Instrument of evaluation[c]	Version	OCPD prevalence range
Cheng et al. 2010	CN	Students	OR	7,675	IPDE	DSM-IV	0.8–1.3
Grant et al. 2004, 2012	US	Community sample of adults	OR	43,093	AUDADIS-IV	DSM-IV	7.7–8.2
Becoña et al. 2013	ES	Community sample of adults	SR	1,081	IPDE	DSM-IV	33.8–39.6
Dereboy et al. 2014	TR	Community sample of adults	SR	774	DIP-Q	DSM-IV	11.7–16.7
Oltmanns et al. 2014	US	Community sample of adults	OR	1,630	SIDP-IV	DSM-IV	2.8–4.7
Gawda and Czubak 2017	PL	General population	OR	1,460	SCID-II	DSM-IV	7.9–11.4
Irfan et al. 2018	PK	Students	OR	1,334	IPDE	DSM-IV	0.002–0.4

[a]AU=Australia; CN=China; DE=Germany; ES=Spain; IS=Iceland; IT=Italy; NO=Norway; PK=Pakistan; PL=Poland; SE=Sweden; TR=Turkey; UK=United Kingdom; US=United States.
[b]OR=observer rated; SR=self-rated.
[c]AUDADIS-IV=Alcohol Use Disorder and Associated Disabilities Interview Schedule—DSM-IV Version; DIP-Q=DSM-IV and ICD-10 Personality Questionnaire; IPDE=International Personality Disorder Examination; PDE=Personality Disorder Examination; PDQ=Personality Diagnostic Questionnaire; SAP=Standardized Assessment of Personality; SCID-II=Structured Clinical Interview for DSM-IV Axis II Personality Disorders; SIDP=Structured Interview for DSM-III Personality Disorders; SIDP-R=Structured Interview for DSM-IV Personality Disorders; SIDP-IV=Structured Interview for DSM-III-R Personality Disorders; SNAP-2=Schedule for Nonadaptive and Adaptive Personality—2nd Edition; SPE=Standardized Psychiatric Examination.

AGE AT ONSET

Although personality disorder by definition is long-standing and pervasive, it is difficult to determine with clarity the usual age at onset of OCPD because of a shortage of prospective studies analyzing the development of personality disorders in youth. Many clinicians are reluctant to diagnose personality disorders in youth, viewing pediatric personality deviations instead as reflective of given developmental stages. However, evidence exists that certain youth are at increased risk for the eventual development of personality disorders as adults (Guilé and Greenfield 2004). A longitudinal study by Bernstein et al. (1993) involving 733 youth ranging in age from 9 to 19 years found the prevalence of OCPD to exceed 13.4%, which is above the prevalence usually seen in adult samples. In another follow-up study, Lewinsohn et al. (1997) reported an 8% prevalence rate of OCPD in young people. Both studies used DSM-III criteria to define OCPD; however, the study by Lewinsohn et al. (1997) required only three diagnostic trait criteria, and therefore the rate may be viewed as inflated. Additional studies suggest that individuals with OCD comorbid with OCPD show a particularly early age at onset of OCD, implying that the psychopathology in the form of OCPD traits starts early in life (Coles et al. 2008; Fineberg et al. 2007).

FAMILY HISTORY

Research with twins suggests that OCPD is highly heritable (Gjerde et al. 2015; Torgersen et al. 2000). Other data suggest that a specific shared heritability exists across OCPD and other OCRDs. For example, OCPD, OCRDs, and autism spectrum disorder cluster not only in the same patients (Hofvander et al. 2009) but also in their family members (Anderluh et al. 2003; Bienvenu et al. 2012; Calvo et al. 2009; Hollander et al. 2003; Nestadt et al. 2000; Özyurt and Besiroglu 2018; Samuels et al. 2000), suggesting that these disorders may share genetic factors in their etiology. In the study by Samuels et al. (2000), the first-degree relatives of probands with OCD showed an increased prevalence of OCPD and high neuroticism scores. In the family study by Calvo et al. (2009), a higher incidence of DSM-IV OCPD was reported in the parents of pediatric OCD probands than in the parents of healthy control children, even after parents with OCD were excluded. In a further study, OCPD was the only personality disorder to co-occur significantly more often in the relatives of OCD probands than in relatives of control subjects after adjusting for OCD in the relatives (Bienvenu et al. 2012). Another family study found that obsessional personality traits may be a specific familial risk factor for anorexia nervosa—an eating disorder with prominent obsessive-compulsive psychopathology (Lilenfeld et al. 1998). Hollander et al. (2003) reported that obsessive-compulsive traits or disorder were more likely to be found in the parents of autistic children if those children showed compulsive behaviors, indicating the possibility that the familial risk shared across OCPD, OCD, and autism spectrum disorder diagnoses relates to the presence of compulsive behavior patterns.

IMPACT

OCPD is associated with significant deficits in interpersonal and intrapersonal function (Cain et al. 2015) and, in the case of psychiatric comorbidity, often predicts a poor response to treatment (see next section). Despite the prevalence of OCPD, however, its impact on psychosocial function remains poorly researched. Existing studies have shown that even after researchers control for comorbid psychiatric disorders, individuals with OCPD show notably high rates of engagement in primary health care use (Sansone et al. 2003, 2004), suggesting that OCPD carries a significant health services burden and cost. For example, compared with patients with major depressive disorder, patients with OCPD were found to be three times as likely to receive psychotherapy (Bender et al. 2001, 2006). Another study found that individuals with OCPD reported comparable impairment in psychosocial functioning and quality of life to those with OCD, one of the most disabling neuropsychiatric disorders (Pinto et al. 2014). A further study in a small sample of patients with OCD found an association between the presence of OCPD and poor social communication, as well as high rates of unemployment, even above that associated with the comorbid OCD (Gadelkarim et al., in press).

Although DSM-III emphasized communication problems, such as the individual's insisting that others submit to his or her way of doing things, which is associated with a lack of awareness of the feelings elicited by this behavior, communication problems are not currently emphasized in the diagnostic descriptions of OCPD. Many clinicians, however, would endorse this as a cardinal feature. Poor social communication may also explain the fact that many people with OCPD find interpersonal relationships difficult (Cain et al. 2015), as well as the high rates of marital disharmony (Reddy and Maitri 2015; Reddy et al. 2016) and of explosive aggressive outbursts (e.g., Villemarette-Pittman et al. 2004). Hoarding is another key OCPD behavior that is likely to have an impact on interpersonal relationships. A better understanding of the nature of these behavioral aspects of OCPD may identify fruitful targets for therapeutic intervention.

COMORBIDITY

The coexistence of two or more illnesses at rates exceeding those expected may be explained by shared etiological (environmental and/or genetic) factors (Fineberg et al. 2007). Several mental disorders are commonly seen in individuals with OCPD. In the McGlashan et al. (2000) Collaborative Longitudinal Personality Disorders Study, performed in a clinical sample of 668 individuals, the most commonly reported diagnoses comorbid with OCPD were major depressive disorder (75.8%), generalized anxiety disorder (29.4%), alcohol abuse/dependence (29.4%), drug abuse/dependence (25.7%), and OCD (20.9%).

Conversely, OCPD rates are elevated in patient groups presenting with other primary psychiatric disorders. For example, OCPD frequently occurs in patients with OCD, with a range from 20% to 34% (Albert et al. 2004; Eisen et al. 2006; Garyfallos et al. 2010; Lochner et al. 2011; Starcevic et al. 2013). OCPD has been found to be more prevalent in patients with early-onset OCD (Pinto et al. 2006). Individuals with OCPD with or without comorbid OCD tend to have poorer mental flexibility on laboratory testing (Fineberg et al. 2007, 2015). Those with comorbid OCD show poorer cognitive-behavioral therapy outcomes, especially when perfectionism is more pronounced (Pinto et al. 2011b), and a greater risk of OCD chronicity (Wewetzer et al. 2001) and relapse (Eisen et al. 2013), suggesting a possible neurodevelopmental etiology for this comorbid subgroup. Indeed, in a recent study of an OCD cohort, OCPD associated strongly with unemployment and with traits of autism spectrum disorder (Gadelkarim et al., in press). However, this study was limited by small size.

Recent studies also indicate that OCPD shows considerable overlap with eating disorders such as anorexia nervosa and binge-eating disorder (Halmi et al. 2005; Kountza et al. 2018). Reported overlap is from 26% to 61% for patients with anorexia nervosa (Anderluh et al. 2003; Kountza et al. 2018) and from 10% to 26% for patients with binge-eating disorder (Friborg et al. 2014; Karwautz et al. 2003). Current research on perfectionism has illustrated its predictive utility in eating disorder symptoms (Ghandour et al. 2018) and has highlighted its association with OCPD (Anderluh et al. 2003; Grilo 2004; von Ranson 2008). Research on personality traits has also indicated perfectionism as a vulnerability factor for body dysmorphic disorder (Buhlmann et al. 2008; Schieber et al. 2013).

OCPD was found to be the most common personality disorder among patients with depressive disorders (30.8%) (Rossi et al. 2001) (see the case vignette at the beginning of this chapter) and, like paranoid personality disorder, is a significant predictor of reduced probability of remission from depression (Agosti et al. 2009). A 6-year prospective study by Grilo et al. (2010) found that patients with OCPD were among those with the highest risk for depressive relapse. OCPD was also found to be the most common personality disorder among patients with bipolar affective disorders (32.4%) (Sjåstad et al. 2012), among elderly individuals with dysthymic disorder (17.1%) (Devanand et al. 2000), and among patients with panic disorder either with agoraphobia (26.7%) (Brooks et al. 1991) or without agoraphobia (11.9%) (Iketani et al. 2002). A study analyzing the association of personality disorders with the prospective 7-year course of anxiety disorders, including aspects of rates of remission, relapse, new episode onset, and chronicity of disorders, found that OCPD diagnosis had negative prognostic significance for generalized anxiety disorder, OCD, and agoraphobia (Ansell et al. 2011). Our preliminary study of patients with anxiety and mood disorders found that the presence of OCPD was related to worse health-related quality of life and perceptions of general health, independent of sociodemographic and clinical characteristics (Gecaite et al. 2018).

OCPD ASSESSMENT

Structured interviews are commonly used to measure OCPD. The most commonly used include the Structured Clinical Interview for DSM-IV Axis II Personality Disorders (SCID-II; First 1997), International Personality Disorder Examination (IPDE; Slade et al. 1998), Structured Interview for DSM-IV Personality (SIDP; Pfohl et al. 1997), and the Diagnostic Interview for Personality Disorders (DIPD; Zanarini et al. 1987). Acceptable interrater reliability is observed in studies using SCID-II, DIPD, and SIDP (Clark and Harrison 2001).

There are no established rating instruments for assessing the severity of OCPD as a whole (Fineberg et al. 2007). However, in several studies, evaluation of individual diagnostic criteria has been used to estimate severity (Ansseau 1996; Calvo et al. 2009; Pinto et al. 2011a). The observer-rated Compulsive Personality Assessment Scale (CPAS; Fineberg et al. 2007) has been partially validated in clinical and community-based samples and translated into various languages (Figure 1–1). CPAS demonstrates face validity, mapping directly on each of the DSM-5 diagnostic criteria for OCPD. It also shows aspects of construct validity: CPAS scores positively correlated with neurocognitive concomitants of OCPD (cognitive inflexibility) in a small community-derived sample (Fineberg et al. 2015) and with clinical factors, including fatigue in patients with mood and anxiety disorders (Burkauskas et al. 2018) and autism spectrum traits in patients with OCD (Gadelkarim et al., in press). Advantages of the CPAS include that it is quick and easy to apply (8 items); it can potentially be adapted as a self-rating instrument; and, because it

Subject's name _____   Date of birth ___ / ___ / ____

Rater's name _____   Date of rating ___ / ___ / ____

Items refer to a stable pattern of enduring traits dating back to adolescence or early adulthood. Use the questions listed as part of a semi-structured interview.

For each item circle the appropriate score:
0 = absent; 1 = mild; 2 = moderate; 3 = severe; 4 = very severe

ITEM	RATING
1. Preoccupation with details Are you preoccupied with details, rules, lists, order, organization or schedules to the extent that the major aim of the activity is lost?	0 1 2 3 4
2. Perfectionism Would you describe yourself as a perfectionist who struggles with completing the task at hand?	0 1 2 3 4
3. Workaholism Are you excessively devoted to work to the exclusion of leisure activities and friendships?	0 1 2 3 4
4. Over-conscientiousness Would you describe yourself as over-conscientious and inflexible about matters of morality, ethics or values?	0 1 2 3 4
5. Hoarding Are you unable to discard worn-out or worthless objects even when they have no sentimental value?	0 1 2 3 4
6. Need for control Are you reluctant to delegate tasks or to work with others unless they submit to exactly your way of doing things?	0 1 2 3 4
7. Miserliness Do you see money as something to be hoarded for future catastrophes?	0 1 2 3 4
8. Rigidity Do you think you are rigid or stubborn?	0 1 2 3 4
Total:	

FIGURE 1–1.   Compulsive Personality Assessment Scale (CPAS).

Source.   Reprinted from Fineberg NA, Sharma P, Sivakumaran T, et al: "Does Obsessive-Compulsive Personality Disorder Belong Within the Obsessive-Compulsive Spectrum?" *CNS Spectrums* 12(6):467–482, 2007. Used with permission.

measures each of the DSM-5 criteria, it can be used to support diagnosis using two approaches: dimensional (each item scored 0–4) and threshold (4 or more items scored ≥3).

The 49-item Pathological Obsessive Compulsive Personality Scale (POPS) is a self-report measure of maladaptive OCPD traits and severity that also has been validated recently (Sadri et al. 2018). It has five subscales: difficulty with change, emotional over-control, rigidity, maladaptive perfectionism, and reluctance to delegate (Pinto et al. 2011a). Self-report versions of OCPD questionnaires could also be derived from larger inventories designed for personality disorder assessment, such as the Millon Clinical Multiaxial Inventory–III (MCMI-III; Millon et al. 1997), SCID-II Personality Questionnaire (SCID-II/PQ), and PDQ (Hyler et al. 1992; Samuel and Widiger 2010). However, these tools may show large variability in their representation of particular diagnostic criteria.

Specific OCPD traits may also be assessed using trait questionnaires, such as the Frost Multidimensional Perfectionism Scales (Stöber 1998), or the Hoarding Rating Scale—Self-Report (Tolin et al. 2008), which is a self-report version of the Hoarding Rating Scale—Interview (Tolin et al. 2010) and is a briefer measure that contains only 5 items, including level of clutter in living spaces, difficulty in discarding possessions, excessive acquisition of items, emotional distress regarding hoarding behavior, and impaired functioning due to hoarding.

All the aforementioned questionnaires still have to be tested for their sensitivity and specificity in capturing DSM-5 OCPD across a broad range of different populations and cultures and in identifying whether these traits are sensitive to change over time—a prerequisite for planning treatment trials.

DIAGNOSTIC EFFICIENCY AND STABILITY

It is recognized that personality disorders represent relatively stable disorders. For example, in the study by Bernstein et al. (1993), young subjects with an initial diagnosis of OCPD were 15 times more likely to be given the same diagnosis 2 years later than were subjects without the initial diagnosis. However, it is also recognized that certain maladaptive traits may improve with the passage of time. Indeed, dimensional evaluation has suggested that OCPD may be characterized by maladaptive trait constellations that are stable in their structure but can change in severity or expression over time (Grilo et al. 2004a).

A study analyzing personality disorder trait stability over time concluded that personality disorders are hybrids of traits and symptomatic behaviors and that the interaction of these elements over time could help to determine the diagnostic stability of a particular personality disorder (McGlashan et al. 2005). An early study investigating the diagnostic efficiency of the criteria required for an OCPD diagnosis found that the presence of three criteria (rigidity and stubbornness, perfectionism, and reluctance to delegate tasks) was generally predictive of the ongoing presence of the diagnosis (Grilo et al. 2001).

In a further longitudinal 24-month follow-up study of OCPD, traits such as preoccupation with details, rigidity and stubbornness, and reluctance to delegate were predictive of primarily stable cases of OCPD (Grilo et al. 2004b). The least prevalent and most changeable criteria in OCPD over the 2-year time period were miserly and strict moral behaviors, suggesting that relatively fixed criteria are more trait-like and attitudinal, whereas the intermittent and reactive criteria are more behavioral. Recent findings have confirmed these results, indicating that rigid perfectionism represents a core trait, expressed in both self-report and clinical interview data in OCPD cases (Liggett and Sellbom 2018).

OCPD may therefore be best conceptualized as a disorder characterized by rigid perfectionism and poor central coherence, with other traits influencing how the disorder manifests in individual cases (Liggett et al. 2018). It has also been noted that a large proportion of OCPD subjects do not remain at the diagnostic threshold for a personality disorder for long and that the average number of criteria present decreases significantly over even just 12 months (Shea et al. 2002). In a blind 24-month reassessment (Grilo et al. 2004b), when evaluated categorically, OCPD rates dropped below diagnostic threshold in 60% of initially diagnosed adult cases, casting question on the usefulness of a categorical method of diagnosis.

THRESHOLD VERSUS DIMENSIONAL MODELS OF OCPD

Within the threshold, or categorical, model of personality disorders, general criteria must be met, including clinically significant distress or impairment in social, occupational, or other domains of functioning. In the case of OCPD, once these general criteria have been met, four or more of the eight listed items are also required to complete the diagnosis as a categorical entity. This model has its challenges because raters often disagree on the number of diagnostic criteria needed (Zanarini et al. 2000). Some authors have suggested that a dimensional model, in which pathological traits are assessed on the basis of their degree of presence (i.e., rather than making a judgment regarding presence or absence), is a more meaningful approach to diagnosis, resulting in higher interrater reliability (Lobbestael et al. 2011; Widiger and Simonsen 2005).

There are various dimensional approaches to personality disorder classification. One of the most established dimensional approaches is the five-factor model (FFM; Bagby and Widiger 2018). A meta-analytic review (Samuel and Widiger 2008) suggested that success in using the FFM as a proxy measure of OCPD depends largely on the questionnaire used. For example, the MCMI-III or the Schedule for Nonadaptive and Adaptive Personality (SNAP) better captures conscientiousness than do the Structured Interview for the Five-Factor Model of Personality (SIFFM) or the NEO Personality Inventory—Revised (NEO PI-R) (Trull and Widiger 1997).

The alternative model for personality disorders presented in DSM-5 Section III, "Emerging Measures and Models," also covers personality disorder function in a dimensional way. This section, however, was included more for research purposes than for clinical use. Thus, the clinical utility of the dimensional models is still under active investigation, and the debate on how best to define DSM OCPD, from a diagnostic standpoint, is yet to be resolved (De Fruyt et al. 2006).

Other dimensional models have been proposed to assess OCPD. One includes dimensions of *perfectionism* (i.e., preoccupation with details, perfectionism, excessive devotion to productivity) and *rigidity* (i.e., rigidity, reluctance to delegate, hypermorality), reflecting underlying interpersonal and intrapersonal control (Ansell et al. 2008). Another dimensional three-factor approach proposes assessing perfectionism, rigidity, and *miserliness* (i.e., miserly spending style, inability to discard) (Grilo et al. 2004b). The upcoming ICD-11 proposes the deletion of all specific types of personality disorders, with the focus placed instead on the severity of disturbances in interpersonal functioning and with specific traits, such as *anankastic*, acting as secondary qualifiers (World Health Organization 2018).

Hypothetically, dimensional OCPD models may be of particular value for translational research aiming to link specific aspects of phenomenology with underpinning neurocognitive substrates because individual traits (or dimensions) may map more closely onto these substrates than does the categorical diagnosis. In addition, because OCPD models allow for measurement of independent dimensions across diverse disorders, they are useful for the transdiagnostic investigation of underpinning neurobiology and treatment targets.

TAKE-HOME POINTS

- OCPD is a common, disabling, and relatively neglected psychiatric disorder.

- OCPD is characterized by stable neurocognitive traits such as perfectionism, rigidity, and a focus on detail, with associated behavioral tendencies—such as behaviors aimed at achieving intrapersonal or interpersonal control, hoarding, and miserliness—that adversely affect psychosocial function and impair quality of life.

- The nosological status of OCPD remains uncertain because the disorder is noted to share diagnostic traits and clinical overlap with certain obsessive-compulsive and related disorders, including OCD, body dysmorphic disorder, and hoarding disorder, and with neurodevelopmental disorders such as autism spectrum disorder.

- Dimensional models for OCPD have been proposed and, if validated, may be of value for translational research into the underpinning biology and treatment.

REFERENCES

Abraham K: Contributions to the theory of anal character, in On Character and Libido Development. Edited by Lewin BD. New York, WW Norton, 1966, pp 165–187

Agosti V, Hellerstein DJ, Stewart JW: Does personality disorder decrease the likelihood of remission in early onset chronic depression? Compr Psychiatry 50(6):491–495, 2009 19840585

Albert U, Maina G, Forner F, et al: DSM-IV obsessive-compulsive personality disorder: prevalence in patients with anxiety disorders and in healthy comparison subjects. Compr Psychiatry 45(5):325–332, 2004 15332194

American Psychiatric Association: Diagnostic and Statistical Manual of Mental Disorders. Washington, DC, American Psychiatric Association, 1952

American Psychiatric Association: Diagnostic and Statistical Manual of Mental Disorders. Washington, DC, American Psychiatric Association, 1968

American Psychiatric Association: Diagnostic and Statistical Manual of Mental Disorders, 3rd Edition. Washington, DC, American Psychiatric Association, 1980

American Psychiatric Association: Diagnostic and Statistical Manual of Mental Disorders, 3rd Edition, Revision. Washington, DC, American Psychiatric Association, 1987

American Psychiatric Association: Diagnostic and Statistical Manual of Mental Disorders, 4th Edition. Washington, DC, American Psychiatric Association, 1994

American Psychiatric Association: Diagnostic and Statistical Manual of Mental Disorders, 4th Edition, Text Revision. Washington, DC, American Psychiatric Association, 2000

American Psychiatric Association: Diagnostic and Statistical Manual of Mental Disorders, 5th Edition. Arlington, VA, American Psychiatric Association, 2013

Anderluh MB, Tchanturia K, Rabe-Hesketh S, et al: Childhood obsessive-compulsive personality traits in adult women with eating disorders: defining a broader eating disorder phenotype. Am J Psychiatry 160(2):242–247, 2003 12562569

Ansell EB, Pinto A, Edelen MO, et al: Structure of Diagnostic and Statistical Manual of Mental Disorders, Fourth Edition criteria for obsessive-compulsive personality disorder in patients with binge eating disorder. Can J Psychiatry 53(12):863–867, 2008 19087485

Ansell EB, Pinto A, Crosby RD, et al: The prevalence and structure of obsessive-compulsive personality disorder in Hispanic psychiatric outpatients. J Behav Ther Exp Psychiatry 41(3):275–281, 2010 20227063

Ansell EB, Pinto A, Edelen MO, et al: The association of personality disorders with the prospective 7-year course of anxiety disorders. Psychol Med 41(5):1019–1028, 2011 20836909

Ansseau M: Serotonergic antidepressants in obsessive personality. Encephale 22:309–310, 1996

Bagby RM, Widiger TA: Five Factor Model personality disorder scales: an introduction to a special section on assessment of maladaptive variants of the Five Factor Model. Psychol Assess 30(1):1–9, 2018 29323509

Becoña E, Fernández del Río E, López-Durán A, et al: Axis II disorders and cigarette smoking among adults from the general population. J Pers Disord 27(3):411–424, 2013 22928853

Bender DS, Dolan RT, Skodol AE, et al: Treatment utilization by patients with personality disorders. Am J Psychiatry 158(2):295–302, 2001 11156814

Bender DS, Skodol AE, Pagano ME, et al: Prospective assessment of treatment use by patients with personality disorders. Psychiatr Serv 57(2):254–257, 2006 16452705

Bernstein DP, Cohen P, Velez CN, et al: Prevalence and stability of the DSM-III-R personality disorders in a community-based survey of adolescents. Am J Psychiatry 150(8):1237–1243, 1993 8328570

Bienvenu OJ, Samuels JF, Wuyek LA, et al: Is obsessive-compulsive disorder an anxiety disorder, and what, if any, are spectrum conditions? A family study perspective. Psychol Med 42(1):1–13, 2012 21733222

Black DW, Noyes R Jr, Pfohl B, et al: Personality disorder in obsessive-compulsive volunteers, well comparison subjects, and their first-degree relatives. Am J Psychiatry 150(8):1226–1232, 1993 8328568

Bodlund O, Ekselius L, Lindström E: Personality traits and disorders among psychiatric outpatients and normal subjects on the basis of the SCID screen questionnaire. Nord J Psychiatry 47:425–433, 1993

Brooks RB, Baltazar PL, McDowell DE, et al: Personality disorders co-occurring with panic disorder with agoraphobia. J Pers Disord 5:328–336, 1991

Buhlmann U, Etcoff NL, Wilhelm S: Facial attractiveness ratings and perfectionism in body dysmorphic disorder and obsessive-compulsive disorder. J Anxiety Disord 22(3):540–547, 2008 17624717

Bulli F, Melli G, Cavalletti V, et al: Comorbid personality disorders in obsessive-compulsive disorder and its symptom dimensions. Psychiatr Q 87(2):365–376, 2016 26442944

Burkauskas J, Fineberg NA, Gecaite J, et al: Obsessive compulsive personality and fatigue in patients with anxiety and mood disorders. Eur Neuropsychopharmacol 28:781–782, 2018

Cain NM, Ansell EB, Simpson HB, et al: Interpersonal functioning in obsessive-compulsive personality disorder. J Pers Assess 97(1):90–99, 2015 25046040

Calvo R, Lázaro L, Castro-Fornieles J, et al: Obsessive-compulsive personality disorder traits and personality dimensions in parents of children with obsessive-compulsive disorder. Eur Psychiatry 24(3):201–206, 2009 19118984

Carter JD, Joyce PR, Mulder RT, et al: Gender differences in the frequency of personality disorders in depressed outpatients. J Pers Disord 13(1):67–74, 1999 10228928

Cheng H, Huang Y, Liu B, et al: Familial aggregation of personality disorder: epidemiological evidence from high school students 18 years and older in Beijing, China. Compr Psychiatry 51(5):524–530, 2010 20728011

Clark LA, Harrison JA: Assessment instruments, in Handbook of Personality Disorders: Theory, Research, and Treatment. Edited by Livesley WJ. New York, Guilford, 2001, pp 277–306

Coid J, Yang M, Tyrer P, et al: Prevalence and correlates of personality disorder in Great Britain. Br J Psychiatry 188:423–431, 2006 16648528

Coles ME, Pinto A, Mancebo MC, et al: OCD with comorbid OCPD: a subtype of OCD? J Psychiatr Res 42(4):289–296, 2008 17382961

Crawford TN, Cohen P, Johnson JG, et al: Self-reported personality disorder in the children in the community sample: convergent and prospective validity in late adolescence and adulthood. J Pers Disord 19(1):30–52, 2005 15899719

De Fruyt F, De Clercq BJ, van de Wiele L, et al: The validity of Cloninger's psychobiological model versus the five-factor model to predict DSM-IV personality disorders in a heterogeneous psychiatric sample: domain facet and residualized facet descriptions. J Pers 74(2):479–510, 2006 16529584

Dereboy C, Güzel HS, Dereboy F, et al: Personality disorders in a community sample in Turkey: prevalence, associated risk factors, temperament and character dimensions. Int J Soc Psychiatry 60(2):139–147, 2014 23396288

Devanand DP, Turret N, Moody BJ, et al: Personality disorders in elderly patients with dysthymic disorder. Am J Geriatr Psychiatry 8(3):188–195, 2000 10910415

Eisen JL, Coles ME, Shea MT, et al: Clarifying the convergence between obsessive compulsive personality disorder criteria and obsessive compulsive disorder. J Pers Disord 20(3):294–305, 2006 16776557

Eisen JL, Sibrava NJ, Boisseau CL, et al: Five-year course of obsessive-compulsive disorder: predictors of remission and relapse. J Clin Psychiatry 74(3):233–239, 2013 23561228

Ekselius L, Tillfors M, Furmark T, et al: Personality disorders in the general population: DSM-IV and ICD-10 defined prevalence as related to sociodemographic profile. Pers Individ Dif 30:311–320, 2001

Fineberg NA, Sharma P, Sivakumaran T, et al: Does obsessive-compulsive personality disorder belong within the obsessive-compulsive spectrum? CNS Spectr 12(6):467–482, 2007 17545957

Fineberg NA, Day GA, de Koenigswarter N, et al: The neuropsychology of obsessive-compulsive personality disorder: a new analysis. CNS Spectr 20(5):490–499, 2015 25776273

First MB: Structured Clinical Interview for DSM-IV Axis II Personality Disorders (SCID-II). Washington, DC, American Psychiatric Press, 1997

Freud S: Character and anal eroticism (1908), in Standard Edition of the Complete Psychological Works of Sigmund Freud, Vol 9. Translated and edited by Strachey J. London, Hogarth Press, 1959, pp 167–176

Friborg O, Martinussen M, Kaiser S, et al: Personality disorders in eating disorder not otherwise specified and binge eating disorder: a meta-analysis of comorbidity studies. J Nerv Ment Dis 202(2):119–125, 2014 24469523

Gadelkarim W, Shahper S, Reid J, et al: Overlap of obsessive-compulsive personality disorder and autism spectrum disorder traits among OCD outpatients: an exploratory study. Int J Psychiatry Clin Pract (in press)

Garyfallos G, Katsigiannopoulos K, Adamopoulou A, et al: Comorbidity of obsessive-compulsive disorder with obsessive-compulsive personality disorder: Does it imply a specific subtype of obsessive-compulsive disorder? Psychiatry Res 177(1–2):156–160, 2010 20163876

Gawda B, Czubak K: Prevalence of personality disorders in a general population among men and women. Psychol Rep 120(3):503–519, 2017 28558606

Gecaite J, Fineberg NA, Juskiene A, et al: Obsessive-compulsive personality is associated with worse health-related quality of life in patients with anxiety and mood disorders. Poster presentation at the International College of Obsessive-Compulsive Spectrum Disorders 14th Annual Scientific Meeting, Barcelona, Spain, October 2018

Ghandour BM, Donner M, Ross-Nash Z, et al: Perfectionism in past and present anorexia nervosa. North American Journal of Psychology 20(3):671–690, 2018

Gjerde LC, Czajkowski N, Røysamb E, et al: A longitudinal, population-based twin study of avoidant and obsessive-compulsive personality disorder traits from early to middle adulthood. Psychol Med 45(16):3539–3548, 2015 26273730

Grant BF, Hasin DS, Stinson FS, et al: Prevalence, correlates, and disability of personality disorders in the United States: results from the National Epidemiologic Survey on Alcohol and Related Conditions. J Clin Psychiatry 65(7):948–958, 2004 15291684

Grant JE, Mooney ME, Kushner MG: Prevalence, correlates, and comorbidity of DSM-IV obsessive-compulsive personality disorder: results from the National Epidemiologic Survey on Alcohol and Related Conditions. J Psychiatr Res 46(4):469–475, 2012 22257387

Grilo CM: Factor structure of DSM-IV criteria for obsessive compulsive personality disorder in patients with binge eating disorder. Acta Psychiatr Scand 109(1):64–69, 2004 14674960

Grilo CM, McGlashan TH, Morey LC, et al: Internal consistency, intercriterion overlap and diagnostic efficiency of criteria sets for DSM-IV schizotypal, borderline, avoidant and obsessive-compulsive personality disorders. Acta Psychiatr Scand 104(4):264–272, 2001 11722301

Grilo CM, Sanislow CA, Gunderson JG, et al: Two-year stability and change of schizotypal, borderline, avoidant, and obsessive-compulsive personality disorders. J Consult Clin Psychol 72(5):767–775, 2004a 15482035

Grilo CM, Skodol AE, Gunderson JG, et al: Longitudinal diagnostic efficiency of DSM-IV criteria for obsessive-compulsive personality disorder: a 2-year prospective study. Acta Psychiatr Scand 110(1):64–68, 2004b 15180781

Grilo CM, Stout RL, Markowitz JC, et al: Personality disorders predict relapse after remission from an episode of major depressive disorder: a 6-year prospective study. J Clin Psychiatry 71(12):1629–1635, 2010 20584514

Guilé JM, Greenfield B: Introduction personality disorders in childhood and adolescence. Can Child Adolesc Psychiatr Rev 13(3):51–52, 2004 19030499

Halmi KA, Tozzi F, Thornton LM, et al: The relation among perfectionism, obsessive-compulsive personality disorder and obsessive-compulsive disorder in individuals with eating disorders. Int J Eat Disord 38(4):371–374, 2005 16231356

Hofvander B, Delorme R, Chaste P, et al: Psychiatric and psychosocial problems in adults with normal-intelligence autism spectrum disorders. BMC Psychiatry 9:35, 2009 19515234

Hollander E, King A, Delaney K, et al: Obsessive-compulsive behaviors in parents of multiplex autism families. Psychiatry Res 117(1):11–16, 2003 12581816

Hyler SE, Skodol AE, Oldham JM, et al: Validity of the Personality Diagnostic Questionnaire–Revised: a replication in an outpatient sample. Compr Psychiatry 33(2):73–77, 1992 1544299

Iketani T, Kiriike N, Stein MB, et al: Relationship between perfectionism, personality disorders and agoraphobia in patients with panic disorder. Acta Psychiatr Scand 106(3):171–178, 2002 12197853

Irfan M, Sethi MR, Abdullah AS, et al: Assessment of personality disorders in students appearing for medical school entrance examination. J Pak Med Assoc 68(12):1763–1768, 2018 30504939

Jackson HJ, Burgess PM: Personality disorders in the community: a report from the Australian National Survey of Mental Health and Wellbeing. Soc Psychiatry Psychiatr Epidemiol 35(12):531–538, 2000 11213842

Janet P: Les Obsessions et la Psychasthenie, 2nd Edition. Paris, Bailliere, 1904

Jones E: Anal-erotic character traits, in Papers on Psychoanalysis, 2nd Edition. London, Bailliere Tindall, 1918

Karwautz A, Troop NA, Rabe-Hesketh S, et al: Personality disorders and personality dimensions in anorexia nervosa. J Pers Disord 17(1):73–85, 2003 12659548

Klein DN, Riso LP, Donaldson SK, et al: Family study of early onset dysthymia: mood and personality disorders in relatives of outpatients with dysthymia and episodic major depression and normal controls. Arch Gen Psychiatry 52(6):487–496, 1995 7771919

Kountza M, Garyfallos G, Ploumpidis D, et al: [The psychiatric comorbidity of anorexia nervosa: A comparative study in a population of French and Greek anorexic patients] [in French]. Encephale 44(5):429–434, 2018 29102367

Kraepelin E, Quen JM: Psychiatry: A Textbook for Students and Physicians, Vol 2. Canton, MA, Science History Publications, 1990

Lenzenweger MF, Loranger AW, Korfine L, et al: Detecting personality disorders in a nonclinical population: application of a 2-stage procedure for case identification. Arch Gen Psychiatry 54(4):345–351, 1997 9107151

Lewinsohn PM, Rohde P, Seeley JR, et al: Axis II psychopathology as a function of Axis I disorders in childhood and adolescence. J Am Acad Child Adolesc Psychiatry 36(12):1752–1759, 1997 9401337

Lewis A: Problems of obsessional illness. Proc R Soc Med 29(4):325–336, 1936 19990606

Liggett J, Sellbom M: Examining the DSM-5 alternative model of personality disorders operationalization of obsessive-compulsive personality disorder in a mental health sample. Pers Disord 9(5):397–407, 2018 29927297

Liggett J, Sellbom M, Bach B: Continuity between DSM-5 Section II and Section III personality traits for obsessive-compulsive personality disorder. Clin Psychol Psychother 25(1):144–151, 2018 29024130

Lilenfeld LR, Kaye WH, Greeno CG, et al: A controlled family study of anorexia nervosa and bulimia nervosa: psychiatric disorders in first-degree relatives and effects of proband comorbidity. Arch Gen Psychiatry 55(7):603–610, 1998 9672050

Lindal E, Stefansson JG: [The prevalence of personality disorders in the greater-Reykjavik area]. Laeknabladid 95(3):179–184, 2009 19318710

Lobbestael J, Leurgans M, Arntz A: Inter-rater reliability of the Structured Clinical Interview for DSM-IV Axis I Disorders (SCID I) and Axis II Disorders (SCID II). Clin Psychol Psychother 18(1):75–79, 2011 20309842

Lochner C, Serebro P, van der Merwe L, et al: Comorbid obsessive-compulsive personality disorder in obsessive-compulsive disorder (OCD): a marker of severity. Prog Neuropsychopharmacol Biol Psychiatry 35(4):1087–1092, 2011 21411045

Maier W, Lichtermann D, Klingler T, et al: Prevalences of personality disorders (DSM-III-R) in the community. J Pers Disord 6:187–196, 1992

McGlashan TH, Grilo CM, Skodol AE, et al: The Collaborative Longitudinal Personality Disorders Study: baseline Axis I/II and II/II diagnostic co-occurrence. Acta Psychiatr Scand 102(4):256–264, 2000 11089725

McGlashan TH, Grilo CM, Sanislow CA, et al: Two-year prevalence and stability of individual DSM-IV criteria for schizotypal, borderline, avoidant, and obsessive-compulsive personality disorders: toward a hybrid model of axis II disorders. Am J Psychiatry 162(5):883–889, 2005 15863789

Millon T, Davis R, Millon C: Millon Clinical Multiaxial Inventory–III. Minneapolis, MN, National Computer Systems, 1997

Moldin SO, Rice JP, Erlenmeyer-Kimling L, et al: Latent structure of DSM-III-R Axis II psychopathology in a normal sample. J Abnorm Psychol 103(2):259–266, 1994 8040495

Moran P, Coffey C, Mann A, et al: Personality and substance use disorders in young adults. Br J Psychiatry 188:374–379, 2006 16582065

Murphy DL, Timpano KR, Wheaton MG, et al: Obsessive-compulsive disorder and its related disorders: a reappraisal of obsessive-compulsive spectrum concepts. Dialogues Clin Neurosci 12(2):131–148, 2010 20623919

Nestadt G, Romanoski AJ, Brown CH, et al: DSM-III compulsive personality disorder: an epidemiological survey. Psychol Med 21(2):461–471, 1991 1876651

Nestadt G, Lan T, Samuels J, et al: Complex segregation analysis provides compelling evidence for a major gene underlying obsessive-compulsive disorder and for heterogeneity by sex. Am J Hum Genet 67(6):1611–1616, 2000 11058433

Oltmanns TF, Rodrigues MM, Weinstein Y, et al: Prevalence of personality disorders at midlife in a community sample: disorders and symptoms reflected in interview, self, and informant reports. J Psychopathol Behav Assess 36(2):177–188, 2014 24954973

Özyurt G, Besiroglu L: Autism spectrum symptoms in children and adolescents with obsessive compulsive disorder and their mothers. Noro Psikiyatri Arsivi 55(1):40–48, 2018 30042640

Pena-Garijo J, Edo Villamón S, Meliá de Alba A, et al: Personality disorders in obsessive-compulsive disorder: a comparative study versus other anxiety disorders. Scientific World Journal 2013:856846, 2013 24453917

Pfohl B, Blum N, Zimmerman M: Structured Interview for DSM-IV Personality (SIDP-IV). Washington, DC, American Psychiatric Publishing, 1997

Pinto A, Mancebo MC, Eisen JL, et al: The Brown Longitudinal Obsessive-Compulsive Study: clinical features and symptoms of the sample at intake. J Clin Psychiatry 67(5):703–711, 2006 16841619

Pinto A, Ansell EB, Wright AGC: A new approach to the assessment of obsessive-compulsive personality. Integrated paper session conducted at the annual meeting of the Society for Personality Assessment. Paper presented at the Annual Meeting of the Society for Personality Assessment, Cambridge, MA, March 2011a

Pinto A, Liebowitz MR, Foa EB, et al: Obsessive compulsive personality disorder as a predictor of exposure and ritual prevention outcome for obsessive compulsive disorder. Behav Res Ther 49(8):453–458, 2011b 21600563

Pinto A, Steinglass JE, Greene AL, et al: Capacity to delay reward differentiates obsessive-compulsive disorder and obsessive-compulsive personality disorder. Biol Psychiatry 75(8):653–659, 2014 24199665

Pitman RK: Janet's Obsessions and Psychasthenia: a synopsis. Psychiatr Q 56(4):291–314, 1984 6399751

Pollak JM: Obsessive-compulsive personality: a review. Psychol Bull 86(2):225–241, 1979 382220

Pollak J: Relationship of obsessive-compulsive personality to obsessive-compulsive disorder: a review of the literature. J Psychol 121(2):137–148, 1987 3585808

Reddy M, Maitri SV: Obsessive-compulsive personality disorder: a case report, in Complicated Cases in Obsessive-Compulsive Disorder. Issue IV: OCD Cases with Poor Insight and Obsessive-Compulsive Personality Disorder. Edited by Reddy MS. New Delhi, India Elsevier, 2015

Reddy MS, Vijay MS, Reddy S: Obsessive-compulsive (anankastic) personality disorder: a poorly researched landscape with significant clinical relevance. Indian J Psychol Med 38(1):1–5, 2016 27011394

Reich J, Yates W, Nduaguba M: Prevalence of DSM-III personality disorders in the community. Soc Psychiatry Psychiatr Epidemiol 24(1):12–16, 1989 2496472

Rossi A, Marinangeli MG, Butti G, et al: Pattern of comorbidity among anxious and odd personality disorders: the case of obsessive-compulsive personality disorder. CNS Spectr 5(9):23–26, 2000 17637577

Rossi A, Marinangeli MG, Butti G, et al: Personality disorders in bipolar and depressive disorders. J Affect Disord 65(1):3–8, 2001 11426507

Sadri SK, McEvoy PM, Pinto A, et al: A psychometric examination of the Pathological Obsessive Compulsive Personality Scale (POPS): initial study in an undergraduate sample. J Pers Assess 1:1–10, 2018 29494778

Samuel DB, Widiger TA: A meta-analytic review of the relationships between the five-factor model and DSM-IV-TR personality disorders: a facet level analysis. Clin Psychol Rev 28(8):1326–1342, 2008 18708274

Samuel DB, Widiger TA: A comparison of obsessive-compulsive personality disorder scales. J Pers Assess 92(3):232–240, 2010 20408023

Samuels JF, Nestadt G, Romanoski AJ, et al: DSM-III personality disorders in the community. Am J Psychiatry 151(7):1055–1062, 1994 8010364

Samuels J, Nestadt G, Bienvenu OJ, et al: Personality disorders and normal personality dimensions in obsessive-compulsive disorder. Br J Psychiatry 177:457–462, 2000 11060001

Samuels J, Eaton WW, Bienvenu OJ 3rd, et al: Prevalence and correlates of personality disorders in a community sample. Br J Psychiatry 180:536–542, 2002 12042233

Sansone RA, Hendricks CM, Sellbom M, et al: Anxiety symptoms and healthcare utilization among a sample of outpatients in an internal medicine clinic. Int J Psychiatry Med 33(2):133–139, 2003 12968826

Sansone RA, Hendricks CM, Gaither GA, et al: Prevalence of anxiety symptoms among a sample of outpatients in an internal medicine clinic: a pilot study. Depress Anxiety 19(2):133–136, 2004 15022149

Schieber K, Kollei I, de Zwaan M, et al: Personality traits as vulnerability factors in body dysmorphic disorder. Psychiatry Res 210(1):242–246, 2013 23890696

Shea MT, Stout R, Gunderson J, et al: Short-term diagnostic stability of schizotypal, borderline, avoidant, and obsessive-compulsive personality disorders. Am J Psychiatry 159(12):2036–2041, 2002 12450953

Sjåstad HN, Gråwe RW, Egeland J: Affective disorders among patients with borderline personality disorder. PloS One 7(12):e50930, 2012 23236411

Slade T, Peters L, Schneiden V, et al: The International Personality Disorder Examination Questionnaire (IPDEQ): preliminary data on its utility as a screener for anxious personality disorder. Int J Methods Psychiatr Res 7:84–88, 1998

Starcevic V, Berle D, Brakoulias V, et al: Obsessive-compulsive personality disorder co-occurring with obsessive-compulsive disorder: conceptual and clinical implications. Aust NZ J Psychiatry 47(1):65–73, 2013 22689335

Stein DJ, Kogan CS, Atmaca M, et al: The classification of obsessive–compulsive and related disorders in the ICD-11. J Affect Disord 190:663–674, 2016 26590514

Stöber J: The Frost Multidimensional Perfectionism Scale revisited: more perfect with four (instead of six) dimensions. Pers Individ Dif 24:481–491, 1998

Stuart S, Pfohl B, Battaglia M, et al: The cooccurrence of DSM-III-R personality disorders. J Pers Disord 12(4):302–315, 1998 9891285

Tolin DF, Frost RO, Steketee G, et al: Family burden of compulsive hoarding: results of an internet survey. Behav Res Ther 46(3):334–344, 2008 18275935

Tolin DF, Frost RO, Steketee G: A brief interview for assessing compulsive hoarding: the Hoarding Rating Scale–Interview. Psychiatry Res 178(1):147–152, 2010 20452042

Torgersen S, Lygren S, Oien PA, et al: A twin study of personality disorders. Compr Psychiatry 41(6):416–425, 2000 11086146

Torgersen S, Kringlen E, Cramer V: The prevalence of personality disorders in a community sample. Arch Gen Psychiatry 58(6):590–596, 2001 11386989

Trull TJ, Widiger TA: Structured Interview for the Five-Factor Model of Personality (SIFFM): Professional Manual. Lutz, FL, Psychological Assessment Resources, 1997

Villemarette-Pittman NR, Stanford MS, Greve KW, et al: Obsessive-compulsive personality disorder and behavioral disinhibition. J Psychol 138(1):5–22, 2004 15098711

Volkert J, Gablonski TC, Rabung S: Prevalence of personality disorders in the general adult population in Western countries: systematic review and meta-analysis. Br J Psychiatry 213(6):709–715, 2018 30261937

von Ranson KM: Personality and eating disorders, in Annual Review of Eating Disorders, Part 2. Edited by Wonderlich S, Mitchell JE, de Zwaan M. Boca Raton, FL, CRC Press, 2008, pp 92–104

Wewetzer C, Jans T, Müller B, et al: Long-term outcome and prognosis of obsessive-compulsive disorder with onset in childhood or adolescence. Eur Child Adolesc Psychiatry 10(1):37–46, 2001 11315534

Wheaton MG, Pinto A: Obsessive-compulsive personality disorder, in The Wiley Handbook of Obsessive-Compulsive Disorders. Edited by Abramowitz JS, McKay D, Storch EA. New York, Wiley, 2017, pp 726–742

Widiger TA, Simonsen E: Alternative dimensional models of personality disorder: finding a common ground. J Pers Disord 19(2):110–130, 2005 15899712

World Health Organization: International Statistical Classification of Diseases and Related Health Problems, 11th Revision (ICD-11) for Mortality and Morbidity Statistics. December 2018. Available at: https://icd.who.int/browse11/l-m/en. Accessed April 5, 2019.

Wu KD, Clark LA, Watson D: Relations between obsessive-compulsive disorder and personality: beyond Axis I-Axis II comorbidity. J Anxiety Disord 20(6):695–717, 2006 16326069

Zanarini MC, Frankenburg FR, Chauncey DL, et al: The Diagnostic Interview for Personality Disorders: interrater and test-retest reliability. Compr Psychiatry 28(6):467–480, 1987 3691072

Zanarini MC, Skodol AE, Bender D, et al: The collaborative longitudinal personality disorders study: Reliability of axis I and II diagnoses. J Pers Disord 14(4):291–299, 2000 11213787

Zhang T, Chow A, Tang Y, et al: Comorbidity of personality disorder in obsessive-compulsive disorder: special emphases on the clinical significance. CNS Spectr 20(5):466–468, 2015 26425800

Zimmerman M, Coryell W: DSM-III personality disorder diagnoses in a nonpatient sample: demographic correlates and comorbidity. Arch Gen Psychiatry 46(8):682–689, 1989 2751402

Zimmerman M, Rothschild L, Chelminski I: The prevalence of DSM-IV personality disorders in psychiatric outpatients. Am J Psychiatry 162(10):1911–1918, 2005 16199838

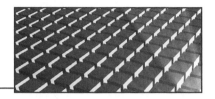

CHAPTER 2

DIAGNOSIS AND CLINICAL FEATURES OF OCPD

Y.C. Janardhan Reddy, M.D.

Case Vignette

Samuel is a 45-year-old university professor in chemistry. He is married and has two children in high school. His main problems are excessive perfectionism, rigidity and stubbornness, preoccupation with details, and inability to delegate responsibility to others; these behaviors have resulted in serious interpersonal problems at work and home and reduced his productivity. His relationship with his children is severely strained because he has no time for them. They describe him as stubborn and very rigid in his thinking. He has not gone on vacation for several years. When he does occasionally take a break from his work, he constantly worries about his pending assignments and fails to enjoy himself. He has unusually high moral standards and tries to impose them on others, including his family and colleagues, and this has further contributed to his problems.

Samuel has always been preoccupied with orderliness and organization; he becomes easily upset if objects in his office, laboratory, or home are moved a bit out of their place. He takes a considerable amount of time in his laboratory every day ordering things his way. He cannot begin work without putting things in his preferred order. After having done that, he has to plan for his day (e.g., planning how to conduct an experiment, researching a topic repeatedly to ensure mistakes are not made) and starts making a list of things to do. However, the most disabling part of his daily routine is his perfectionism. He has to be perfect in everything he does, including his work; he pays attention to minor details, worries that he may not have done a task to perfection, and keeps going over the same things again and again to make sure that everything is done to his level of perfection. Others find his perfectionism to be excessive and to interfere in task completion.

As a result of this behavior, Samuel does not complete most of his research assignments on time, keeps procrastinating, and misses deadlines. He insists that his students conduct experiments and write papers exactly his way. His students have been unable to complete their courses on time because of his insistence on their doing things perfectly. He takes an inordinately long time to complete a research paper because he becomes preoccupied with minor details and revises repeatedly to make sure there are no errors of commission or omission. He takes 30 minutes to draft an e-mail that can be written in 5 minutes because he strives to make sure that the language is perfect and the matter is conveyed exactly as he intends. He finds it very difficult to delegate work to his colleagues and students. He prefers doing things himself lest others make mistakes.

Obsessive-compulsive personality disorder (OCPD) or anankastic personality disorder is the most common personality disorder in the general population (de Reus and Emmelkamp 2012; Grant et al. 2012), with a lifetime prevalence of 3%–9% (Albert et al. 2004; Grant et al. 2012; Samuels et al. 2000). It is associated with psychosocial dysfunction (Mancebo et al. 2005; Pinto et al. 2014; Skodol et al. 2002) and reduced quality of life (Mancebo et al. 2005; Pinto et al. 2014). It is highly comorbid with other psychiatric disorders (Diedrich and Voderholzer 2015), particularly obsessive-compulsive disorder (OCD) (Coles et al. 2008; Pinto et al. 2006; Samuels et al. 2000), body dysmorphic disorder (Phillips and McElroy 2000; Veale et al. 1996), and eating disorders (Anderluh et al. 2003; Nilsson et al. 1999). In this chapter, clinical features of OCPD are discussed, including evolution of diagnostic criteria and the criteria recommended in the latest versions of the American Psychiatric Association's *Diagnostic and Statistical Manual of Mental Disorders* (DSM) and the World Health Organization's *International Classification of Diseases* (ICD).

NOSOLOGY OF OCPD

As defined in DSM-IV (American Psychiatric Association 1994), DSM-5 (American Psychiatric Association 2013), and ICD-10 (World Health Organization 1992), OCPD is a disorder characterized by preoccupation with orderliness, perfectionism, and behavioral and mental interpersonal control, at the expense of flexibility, openness, and efficiency. It has an onset in childhood or adolescence and tends to manifest in a variety of contexts. Although the classificatory systems seem to have certain common core features, they do differ substantially.

CATEGORICAL CLASSIFICATION OF OCPD

DSM

OCPD is one of the few personality disorders described in all versions of DSM, from DSM-I to DSM-5. In DSM-I (American Psychiatric Association 1952), *compulsive personality* was described as follows:

> Such individuals are characterized by chronic, excessive, or obsessive concern with adherence to standards of conscience or of conformity. They may be overinhibited, overconscientious, and may have an inordinate capacity for work. Typically, they are rigid and lack a normal capacity for relaxation. (p. 37)

It was seen as a reaction that "may appear as a persistence of an adolescent pattern of behavior, or as a regression from more mature functioning as a result of stress" (American Psychiatric Association 1952, p. 37).

In DSM-II (American Psychiatric Association 1968), the name was changed to *obsessive-compulsive personality*, and the term *anankastic personality* was introduced. In DSM-III (American Psychiatric Association 1980), affective constriction and difficulty in expressing tender and warm emotions were included in the criteria for the first time. In DSM-IV (American Psychiatric Association 1994) and DSM-5 (American Psychiatric Association 2013), which have almost identical descriptions of OCPD, the DSM-III criteria pertaining to affect were downplayed, but additional criteria were added, such as excessive devotion to work and productivity to the exclusion of leisure, overconscientiousness, miserliness, and difficulty in discarding worthless items. The DSM-5 diagnostic criteria for OCPD (American Psychiatric Association 2013) are shown in Box 2–1 (American Psychiatric Association 2013).

The DSM approach to the diagnosis of OCPD has been criticized because of problems of specificity (ability to identify correctly individuals who do not have OCPD) due to a polythetic approach, sensitivity (ability to identify correctly all those with OCPD), and poor psychometric properties (Farmer and Chapman 2002; Fossati et al. 2006; Hertler 2013; Hummelen et al. 2008; Samuel and Widiger 2011). According to DSM-IV and DSM-5, a diagnosis of OCPD can be made if four of the eight criteria are present; this essentially means that two different people with a

---

BOX 2–1.   DSM-5 diagnostic criteria for obsessive-compulsive
            personality disorder

A pervasive pattern of preoccupation with orderliness, perfectionism, and mental and interpersonal control, at the expense of flexibility, openness, and efficiency, beginning by early adulthood and present in a variety of contexts, as indicated by four (or more) of the following:

1. Is preoccupied with details, rules, lists, order, organization, or schedules to the extent that the major point of the activity is lost.
2. Shows perfectionism that interferes with task completion (e.g., is unable to complete a project because his or her own overly strict standards are not met).
3. Is excessively devoted to work and productivity to the exclusion of leisure activities and friendships (not accounted for by obvious economic necessity).
4. Is overconscientious, scrupulous, and inflexible about matters of morality, ethics, or values (not accounted for by cultural or religious identification).
5. Is unable to discard worn-out or worthless objects even when they have no sentimental value.
6. Is reluctant to delegate tasks or to work with others unless they submit to exactly his or her way of doing things.
7. Adopts a miserly spending style toward both self and others; money is viewed as something to be hoarded for future catastrophes.
8. Shows rigidity and stubbornness.

Source.   Reprinted from American Psychiatric Association: *Diagnostic and Statistical Manual of Mental Disorders,* 5th Edition. Arlington, VA, American Psychiatric Association, 2013, pp. 678–679. Copyright © 2013 American Psychiatric Association. Used with permission.

diagnosis of OCPD can have entirely different sets of symptoms, bringing in the plurality of types.

There has been considerable debate as to which are the core features of OCPD. In a large multisite study of the course and stability of the DSM-IV personality disorders, four of the OCPD criteria—preoccupied with details, perfectionism, reluctance to delegate, and rigid and stubborn—were found to be useful for making a diagnosis of OCPD (Grilo et al. 2001), and the last three of these were also the most stable over the 2-year follow-up period (McGlashan et al. 2005). Other symptoms such as miserliness, workaholic behavior, and hoarding have been found to be unsatisfactory for making a diagnosis of OCPD (Grilo et al. 2001; Hummelen et al. 2008). Overconscientiousness is considered to be the defining feature of OCPD from which other symptoms seem to manifest (Samuel and Widiger 2011), but OCPD can now be diagnosed without it

The problems of sensitivity include exclusion of essential features of OCPD, such as problems in future-oriented planning, attentional bias to minute details, affect dysregulation, and inclusion of certain features such as miserliness and hoarding (Fossati et al. 2006; Hertler 2013; Hummelen et al. 2008; Riddle et al. 2016). In DSM-5, hoarding is included in criteria sets for OCPD, OCD (when secondary to obsessions), and hoarding disorder (American Psychiatric Association 2013).

ICD

The diagnostic criteria for anankastic personality disorder in ICD-10 (Table 2–1) are similar to those for OCPD in DSM-IV and DSM-5 but with some differences. Whereas DSM includes miserliness and hoarding, which are perhaps not the core features of OCPD (Fineberg et al. 2014), ICD-10 includes insistent and unwelcome intrusions and feelings of excessive doubt and concern, which are typical of OCPD as well as OCD and anxiety disorders.

DIMENSIONAL MODELS OF OCPD

A categorical approach adopted in the various versions of DSM and in ICD-10 assumes that the personality disorders are distinct from each other and that they are unidimensional, but the empirical literature suggests otherwise (Ansell et al. 2008; Grilo 2004; Riddle et al. 2016; Sanislow et al. 2002). The dimensional approach posits that personality disorder traits merge imperceptibly into normality and into one another (O'Connor 2005). In fact, most of the traits of OCPD are maladaptive variants of general personality functioning (Widiger et al. 2002). Although categorical diagnoses have clinical utility, dimensional approaches may provide greater insight into the biological substrates (Riddle et al. 2016).

In studies of OCPD and comorbid eating disorder, either a two-factor model (Ansell et al. 2008) or a three-factor model (Grilo 2004) better explained OCPD. In a factor analytical study of the eight DSM-IV OCPD criteria plus indecision, the OCD Collaborative Genetics Study group identified two dimensions of OCPD: 1) order/control, including perfectionism, excessive devotion to work, overconscientiousness, reluctance to delegate, and rigidity, and 2) hoarding/indecision, including inability to discard and indecisiveness (Riddle et al. 2016). The first dimension is similar to the rigid perfectionism described in the DSM-5 alternative model (see next paragraph) and includes five of the eight

---

TABLE 2–1. ICD-10 diagnostic criteria for anankastic personality disorder

---

General criteria for personality disorder should be met and at least four of the following must be present:

1. Feelings of excessive doubt and caution

2. Preoccupation with details, rules, lists, order, organization, or schedule

3. Perfectionism that interferes with task completion

4. Excessive conscientiousness and scrupulousness and undue preoccupation with productivity to the exclusion of pleasure and interpersonal relationships[a]

5. Excessive pedantry and adherence to social conventions

6. Rigidity and stubbornness

7. Unreasonable insistence that others submit to exactly his or her way of doing things, or unreasonable reluctance to allow others to do things

8. Intrusion of insistent and unwelcome thoughts or impulses[b]

---

[a]This criterion was split into two separate criteria (excessive conscientiousness and undue preoccupation with productivity) in the Diagnostic Criteria for Research.
[b]This criterion was removed in the Diagnostic Criteria for Research and is present only in the clinical guidelines.
Source. Reprinted from World Health Organization: *The ICD-10 Classification of Mental and Behavioural Disorders: Clinical Descriptions and Diagnostic Guidelines.* Geneva, World Health Organization, 1992, p. 127 (F60.5, anankastic personality disorder). Available at: https://apps.who.int/iris/bitstream/handle/10665/37108/9241544554.pdf. Used with permission.

symptoms of the official definition of OCPD, whereas the second dimension has core features of hoarding disorder in addition to indecisiveness, one of six associated features supporting diagnosis listed in DSM-5 for hoarding disorder. Preoccupation with details loaded on both factors at a level just below the cutoff criterion for inclusion, whereas miserliness loaded on the hoarding dimension only but below the cutoff for inclusion. It appears that miserliness and hoarding are probably not essential features of OCPD, and indecision is associated more with hoarding. Including miserliness and hoarding in the description of OCPD might add to the heterogeneity of the OCPD construct.

DSM-5

DSM-5 includes an alternative set of criteria for the personality disorders (placed in Section III, "Emerging Measures and Models") that is informed by the five-factor model (FFM; Costa and McCrae 1992). It is a combination of both dimensional and categorical approaches. The criteria for OCPD diagnosis using this approach are the following: 1) at least moderate level of impairment in personality functioning in at least two of four areas (identity, self-direction, empathy, and intimacy) and 2) in addition to rigid perfectionism (an essential criterion), at least two of three additional features: perseveration, intimacy avoidance, and restricted affectivity. The DSM-5 alternative model criteria for OCPD are shown in Box 2–2.

Although DSM-5 has introduced a hybrid alternative model combining categorical and dimensional approaches, the official criteria and the alternative model differ in many ways, resulting in a lack of congruity within the same classificatory system. First, a diagnosis of OCPD (see DSM-5, Section II, "Diagnostic Criteria and Codes") has a polythetic approach and requires any four of the eight criteria, whereas the alternative approach (see DSM-5, Section III) has a hierarchical approach in that rigid perfectionism is an essential criterion. Second, two official criteria, miserliness and inability to discard objects (hoarding), are absent in the alternative criteria, and the alternative criteria include four areas that are not part of the official criteria: avoidance of intimacy, perseveration, difficulty in empathizing with others, and constricted affect. Although data supporting inclusion of miserliness and hoarding as features of OCPD are insufficient (Grilo et al. 2001; Hummelen et al. 2008; Riddle et al. 2016), the alternative criteria have brought back constricted affect in the description of OCPD; this criterion was initially part of the DSM-III and DSM-III-R criteria but was excluded in DSM-IV and DSM-5. Third, the official diagnosis of OCPD has a categorical approach, whereas the alternative approach combines categorical and dimensional approaches. Fourth, the official criteria may lead to overdiagnosis of OCPD, but the alternative criteria are strict and hierarchical, resulting in less frequent diagnoses of OCPD. Individuals who are diagnosed with OCPD using the official criteria may not get the same diagnosis with the alternative criteria, and vice versa. This lack of clarity on the core features of OCPD may lead not only to greater heterogeneity of OCPD but also to difficulty in integrating research findings.

ICD-11

The approach to classification of personality disorders in ICD-11 reflects a significant departure from that in DSM and ICD-10 in that the categorical system of classifying personality disorders is completely replaced by a dimensional approach (Tyrer et al. 2011, 2015), which aligns with other dimensional schemes such as the five-factor model (Mulder et al. 2011; Oltmanns and Widiger 2018; Widiger and Mullins-Sweatt 2010; Widiger and Simonsen 2005) and the DSM-5 alternative model of personality disorders (American Psychiatric Association 2013; Bach et al. 2018; Lotfi et al. 2018). Three steps are involved in the classification of personality disorders in ICD-11: 1) determining whether general diagnostic requirements for personality disorders are satisfied; 2) grading

---

BOX 2–2.   Proposed diagnostic criteria for obsessive-compulsive
personality disorder in the alternative DSM-5 model

A. Moderate or greater impairment in personality functioning, manifested by characteristic difficulties in two or more of the following four areas:

  1. *Identity:* Sense of self derived predominantly from work or productivity; constricted experience and expression of strong emotions.
  2. *Self-direction:* Difficulty completing tasks and realizing goals, associated with rigid and unreasonably high and inflexible internal standards of behavior; overly conscientious and moralistic attitudes.
  3. *Empathy:* Difficulty understanding and appreciating the ideas, feelings, or behaviors of others.
  4. *Intimacy:* Relationships seen as secondary to work and productivity; rigidity and stubbornness negatively affect relationships with others.

B. Three or more of the following four pathological personality traits, one of which must be (1) Rigid perfectionism:

  1. *Rigid perfectionism* (an aspect of extreme Conscientiousness [the opposite pole of Disinhibition]): Rigid insistence on everything being flawless, perfect, and without errors or faults, including one's own and others' performance; sacrificing of timeliness to ensure correctness in every detail; believing that there is only one right way to do things; difficulty changing ideas and/or viewpoint; preoccupation with details, organization, and order.
  2. *Perseveration* (an aspect of **Negative Affectivity**): Persistence at tasks long after the behavior has ceased to be functional or effective; continuance of the same behavior despite repeated failures.
  3. *Intimacy avoidance* (an aspect of **Detachment**): Avoidance of close or romantic relationships, interpersonal attachments, and intimate sexual relationships.
  4. *Restricted affectivity* (an aspect of **Detachment**): Little reaction to emotionally arousing situations; constricted emotional experience and expression; indifference or coldness.

Source.   Reprinted from American Psychiatric Association: *Diagnostic and Statistical Manual of Mental Disorders,* 5th Edition. Arlington, VA, American Psychiatric Association, 2013, pp. 768–769. Copyright © 2013 American Psychiatric Association. Used with permission.

the severity of personality disorder as personality difficulty, mild personality disorder, moderate personality disorder, or severe personality disorder; and 3) considering which of five trait domain qualifiers (negative affectivity, detachment, dissociality, disinhibition, and anankastia) are applicable (Bach and First 2018; Farnam and Zamanlu 2018). The clinician can also use two additional qualifiers: personality difficulty and borderline personality. Severity of personality functioning is determined by the extent of disturbances in aspects of the self (e.g., sense of identity, self-worth, self-direction); interpersonal dysfunction (e.g., interpersonal relationships, empathy); and emotional (e.g., appropriate emotional experience and expression), cognitive (e.g., accuracy of interpersonal appraisals, decision making, appropriate stability and flexibility of belief systems), and behavioral (e.g., impulsivity, propensity to self-harm) manifestations of dysfunction (Bach and First 2018). Classifying personality disorders on the basis of severity is expected to inform prognosis and intensity of treatment, whereas trait qualifiers may help in choosing specific treatment (Bach and First 2018).

The ICD-11 dimensional approach to classification of personality disorders is very similar to the alternative model of personality disorder in DSM-5. It allows a cross-walk with the DSM-5 alternative model using the measures employed to diagnose personality disorders in DSM-5 (Bach and First 2018). However, anankastia is included as a trait qualifier in ICD-11 but not in DSM-5, and psychoticism is included in DSM-5 but not in ICD-11. ICD-11 defines *anankastia* as "a narrow focus on one's rigid standard of perfection and of right and wrong, and on controlling one's own and others' behavior and controlling situations to ensure conformity to these standards" (World Health Organization 2019, p. 178). Common manifestations of anankastia, not all of which may be present in an individual, include perfectionism, preoccupation with details, overconscientiousness, difficulty in delegating responsibilities to others, hyperscheduling and excessive planning, undue orderliness, emotional restriction, rigidity and stubbornness, and perseveration. In a recent study, Bach et al. (2018) examined the association between ICD-11 and DSM-5 trait domains, simultaneously with the DSM-IV categorical diagnoses, in a sample of 226 psychiatric outpatients and found that both models capture substantial information and showed continuity with categorical personality disorders. ICD-11 was superior in capturing OCPD, whereas DSM-5 was superior in capturing schizotypal personality disorder. These findings suggest that a cross-walk is possible between categorical and dimensional models without losing much information.

ASSESSMENT OF OCPD

It is evident that the conceptualization of OCPD has changed over the years, and there is no clear consensus on its core features. Its criteria sets have been subject to periodic modifications, and with the introduction of dimensional approaches in DSM-5 and ICD-11, the need for psychometrically valid instruments that assess both categorical and trait features of personality disorders including OCPD has only increased. Here, we briefly mention instruments that have been used commonly in clinical practice and research (for an exhaustive review, see Furnham et al. 2014).

There are several structured interviews for diagnosing all personality disorders, including OCPD. Notable among them are the Structured Clinical Interview for DSM-5 Personality Disorders (SCID-5-PD; First et al. 2015), the Diagnostic Interview for DSM-IV Personality Disorders (DIPD-IV; Zanarini et al. 1996), the Personality Disorder Interview (PDI; Widiger et al. 1995), and the International Personality Disorder Examination (IPDE; Loranger 1999). The SCID-5-PD is a semistructured diagnostic interview for clinicians and researchers that assesses the 10 DSM-5 personality disorders and has an optional self-report screening instrument, the Structured Clinical Interview for DSM-5 Screening Personality Questionnaire (SCID-5-SPQ; M.B. First et al. 2016). The SCID-5-SPQ helps to reduce the time of the SCID-5-PD interview. The IPDE is another widely used structured interview that assesses personality disorders across both DSM-IV and ICD-10. The IPDE Questionnaire is a screening tool to be used alongside the IPDE (Loranger 1999).

Commonly used self-rating scales are the Personality Diagnostic Questionnaire–4 (PDQ-4; Hyler 1994), Millon Clinical Multiaxial Inventory–III (MCMI-III; Millon et al. 1997), Minnesota Multiphasic Personality Inventory–2 (MMPI-2; Butcher et al. 1989), OMNI Personality Inventory (OMNI; Loranger 2002), Wisconsin Personality Disorders Inventory–IV (WISPI-IV; Klein and Benjamin 1996), and Schedule for Nonadaptive and Adaptive Personality (SNAP; Clark 1993). All these inventories include varying numbers of items covering OCPD. For an extensive review of these scales, the reader may refer to previous publications on the topic (Furnham et al. 2014; Samuel and Widiger 2010; Widiger and Boyd 2009). The Pathological Obsessive Compulsive Personality Scale (POPS; Sadri et al. 2018) and the Clinical Perfectionism Questionnaire (CPQ; Stoeber and Damian 2014) specifically assess OCPD traits.

The Five Factor Obsessive-Compulsive Inventory (FFOCI; Samuel et al. 2012) has 12 scales that measure various aspects of OCPD from the perspective of the FFM. The inventory has demonstrated good convergent and discriminant validity with established measures of the OCPD and the FFM facets. A shorter version of the FFOCI is also available as a briefer measure of the OCPD traits (Griffin et al. 2018). The Structured Clinical Interview for the DSM-5 Alternative Model for Personality Disorders (SCID-5-AMPD) has three modules: Module I is devoted to the dimensional assessment of self and interpersonal functioning using the Level of Personality Functioning Scale (First et al. 2018a), and Module II assesses the five trait domains and their corresponding 25 trait facets (Skodol et al. 2018). Module III, which can be used independently or in combination with either of the other two modules, provides a comprehensive assessment of six specific personality disorders, including OCPD (First et al. 2018b).

Via cross-walk, SCID-5-AMPD Modules I and II can be used to generate ICD-11 severity of personality dysfunction and trait domain qualifiers, respectively (Bach and First 2018). Self-report measures can also be used to assess severity of personality dysfunction and trait qualifiers. The Level of Personality Functioning Scale—Brief Form 2.0 (LPFS-BF) also measures impairment of self and interpersonal functioning and is consistent with the ICD-11 severity classification (Bach and Anderson 2018; Bach and Hutsebaut 2018). The Personality Inventory for the DSM-5 (PID-5) can also help derive ICD-11 trait domain qualifiers (Bach et al. 2017). A 60-item self-report or informant-report instrument called the Personality Inventory for the ICD-11 (PiCD) also describes the five ICD-11 trait domains (Oltmanns and Widiger 2018).

CLINICAL FEATURES OF OCPD

Features of OCPD across classificatory systems, including the alternative model of DSM-5 and the dimensional approach of ICD-11 (World Health Organization 2019), are compared in Table 2–2. It is also important to differentiate OCPD from OCD because they are often comorbid with each other and have similar clinical presentations.

It is common in clinical practice to distinguish OCPD from OCD by the absence of typical obsessions/compulsions and ego-dystonicity. Differences in the phenomenology of OCD and OCPD are summarized in Table 2–3, but these are rather broad differences that help to distinguish one from the other. There is also considerable overlap in the phenomenology of the disorders. For example, perfectionism in OCPD is not always ego-syntonic; many individuals with OCPD are distressed about being unduly perfectionistic because it interferes with task completion. Similarly, fears of contamination and the washing and cleaning compulsions are not always perceived as excessive or irrational and are often not resisted.

Recently, there has been a great interest in sensory phenomena in OCD. A sense of "incompleteness" and "just-right" phenomena are known to underlie many symptoms, such as symmetry, counting, repeating, and slowness (Summerfeldt 2004). These phenomena are also known to contribute to perfectionism in OCPD (Ecker et al. 2014; Sum-

TABLE 2–2. Obsessive-compulsive personality disorder traits in classificatory systems

Criteria	DSM-III	DSM-III-R	DSM-IV	DSM-5	DSM-5 alternative model	ICD-10	ICD-11 anankastia
Excessive preoccupation with order, rules, lists, and details		✓	✓	✓		✓	✓
Rigid perfectionism	✓	✓	✓	✓	✓	✓	✓
Workaholism (to the exclusion of leisure and family and friends)	✓	✓	✓	✓	✓	✓	
Overconscientiousness, scrupulousness, or inflexibility about morality and ethics		✓	✓	✓	✓	✓	✓
Reluctance to delegate responsibility or tasks to others	✓	✓	✓	✓	✓	✓	✓
Rigidity and stubbornness			✓	✓	✓	✓	✓
Restricted affective experience and expression	✓	✓			✓	✓	✓

TABLE 2–2. Obsessive-compulsive personality disorder traits in classificatory systems *(continued)*

Criteria	DSM-III	DSM-III-R	DSM-IV	DSM-5	DSM-5 alternative model	ICD-10	ICD-11 anankastia
Difficulty in empathizing with others					✓		
Perseveration					✓		✓
Avoidance of intimacy					✓		✓
Indecisiveness	✓	✓					
Hoarding		✓	✓	✓			
Miserliness		✓	✓	✓			
Excessive doubt and caution						✓	
Excessive pedantry and adherence to social norms						✓	
Intrusive unwelcome thoughts or impulses						✓	

TABLE 2–3. Phenomenology of obsessive-compulsive personality
           disorder (OCPD) and obsessive-compulsive disorder (OCD)

OCPD	OCD
Traits are mostly ego-syntonic, consistent with the individual's belief system, which is viewed as reasonable.	Obsessions are intrusive, mostly ego-dystonic, and viewed as irrational/excessive/ unwanted.
	Compulsions are often performed in response to obsessions or according to rules; they are perceived as excessive and not connected in a realistic way with what they intend to prevent or neutralize.
The individual offers no inner resistance.	The individual offers resistance and tries to control obsessions and compulsions.
Insight is generally poor.	Insight is generally well preserved.
The individual insists on "doing things my way, the right way."	The individual experiences anxiety about feared consequences.
Perfectionism is global and involves all spheres.	Perfectionism or rules are focal and limited to feared events or specific compulsive behaviors.
A sense of "incompleteness" can contribute to perfectionism and indecisiveness.	A sense of "incompleteness" or something being "just not right" is common and may contribute to symmetry, counting, repeating, and slowness.
The individual has difficulty discarding worn-out or worthless objects even when they do not have sentimental value because "you never know when you might need it."[a]	Hoarding is secondary to other typical obsessions and compulsions and not because of any utilitarian value.

[a]This feature overlaps with DSM-5 hoarding disorder and, interestingly, is not a feature of the ICD-10 anankastic personality disorder or the DSM-5 alternative model.

merfeldt et al. 2000). Although some degree of overlap between OCPD and OCD is perhaps inevitable, similar diagnostic criteria for OCPD and OCD may also contribute to spurious overlap. Hoarding is a symptom of OCPD in both DSM-IV and DSM-5. In DSM-IV, there is no hoarding disorder, and hoarding is recognized as a symptom of OCD. In DSM-5, there is a separate hoarding disorder, but hoarding secondary to obsessions and compulsions can lead to diagnostic confusion if the phenomena are not properly evaluated. Similarly, perfectionism is one of the key characteristics of OCPD and may contribute to overlap with OCD when perfectionism contributes to symmetry, ordering, arranging, and repeating compulsions (Starcevic and Brakoulias 2014).

On the basis of review of the extant literature, the following seem to be some core features of OCPD. They are discussed in relation to Samuel, introduced in the case vignette at the beginning of this chapter. Samuel was evaluated using the SCID-5-PD and exhibited six of the eight diagnostic criteria for DSM-5 OCPD.

1. *Rigid perfectionism:* Undue perfectionism is one of the core features of OCPD. The perfectionism is self-imposed and set at an unusually high standard to the extent that it impairs task completion. Attention is paid to minute and often irrelevant and peripheral details at the expense of completing an activity on time. For example, Samuel cannot complete his research projects and scientific papers because he has to do them "perfectly" his way and he goes over experiments and papers again and again to make sure there are no errors. This annoys others, and he hardly ever completes his projects on time. In essence, he has disabling perfectionism.

2. *Preoccupation with details, order, and organization:* Individuals with OCPD often tend to achieve a sense of control or mastery through painstaking attention to rules, lists, order, organization, and schedules. They tend to be overcautious, pay attention to trivial details and procedures, and spend inordinate amounts of time planning and organizing to the extent that the intended activity does not get completed. They tend to be oblivious to the fact that others become annoyed by their delays. Samuel spends considerable amounts of time in his workplace trying to be orderly. He cannot start an activity without an elaborate plan and making a list of things to do. Unfortunately, this orderliness is followed by disabling perfectionism, and together they contribute to significant dysfunction and inefficiency.

3. *Excessive devotion to work:* Individuals with OCPD devote excessive time to work and productivity at the cost of personal leisure and family and social commitments; they are often described as workaholics. They cannot find time to relax or take a weekend day off. They often do not take vacations, or they keep postponing pleasur-

able activities. Even if they do take a vacation, they carry work with them (e.g., spending time on a laptop doing work-related tasks) and participate in leisure activities as if these activities are other tasks that need to be performed in an organized manner. Samuel's devotion to work at the expense of his leisure activities and family commitments is an example of this trait.

4. *Reluctance to delegate:* Individuals with OCPD often have difficulty delegating work to others because they have no confidence that other people can do tasks or work in the correct way. They feel that others may make mistakes or not do assignments the way they should be done. For them, there is only one way of doing things correctly: their own way. They have a tendency to give elaborate instructions to others about the nature of work assigned to them and are often unhappy that things are not done to their satisfaction. This applies not only to work at the office but also to activities at home—there is only one correct way to dry clothes, wash dishes, iron clothes, and so forth.

5. *Overconscientiousness and inflexibility with matters of morality, values, and ethics:* Individuals with OCPD force on themselves and impose on others their rigid value system and principles. They rigidly follow all rules and regulations and refuse to bend rules in any circumstances. Samuel has this trait, which has resulted in severe interpersonal issues with family members and colleagues.

6. *Rigidity and stubbornness:* Individuals with OCPD want everything their way; there is only one "correct" way. They have great difficulty in seeing others' viewpoints and do not budge easily or accept others' perspectives. This rigidity in thinking and stubbornness can lead to serious interpersonal issues with others. This is another of the typical features of OCPD that Samuel exhibits.

Although hoarding and miserliness are described in DSM-5 OCPD, there is insufficient evidence to consider them as essential features of OCPD, and Samuel does not seem to demonstrate these features.

CONCLUSION

OCPD is marked by the core feature of extreme conscientiousness that manifests itself as perfectionism, rigidity and stubbornness in thinking, preoccupation with details, difficulty in delegating responsibility to others, and excessive devotion to work and productivity. However, the concept of and criteria to diagnose OCPD have changed over time with additions to, subtractions from, and modifications of the classificatory systems. Recently, there has been renewed interest in understanding personality disorders from a dimensional perspective. Nonetheless, the categorical diagnoses continue to exist because of their clinical utility and because of want of additional research on clinical and research utility of dimensional classification. The dimensional approach in DSM-5 and ICD-11 may boost research on a dimensional perspective of OCPD.

TAKE-HOME POINTS

- OCPD is a common personality disorder characterized by excessive perfectionism, overconscientiousness, and rigidity in thinking.

- Miserliness and hoarding are symptoms of DSM-5 OCPD, but there is insufficient evidence to include them as core features of OCPD.

- An accurate diagnosis of OCPD may require a detailed clinical assessment, preferably using a structured or a semistructured interview.

- Although OCPD and OCD have phenomenological similarity, OCPD is characterized by ego-syntonic traits with poorer insight and less inner resistance and by absence of the classical obsessions and compulsions typical of OCD.

- The DSM-5 OCPD criteria and the proposed criteria for OCPD in the DSM-5 alternative model are not congruent with each other. The official criteria follow the traditional polythetic approach, whereas the alternative criteria for OCPD are hierarchical and are a combination of both categorical and dimensional approaches. This incongruent approach may contribute to heterogeneity in the concept of OCPD, which in turn may result in difficulty in integrating research findings.

- Classification of personality disorders in ICD-11 has undergone a major paradigmatic shift in that categorical diagnoses have been eliminated, but the trait qualifier anankastia is similar to other descriptions of OCPD.

REFERENCES

Albert U, Maina G, Forner F, et al: DSM-IV obsessive-compulsive personality disorder: prevalence in patients with anxiety disorders and in healthy comparison subjects. Compr Psychiatry 45(5):325–332, 2004 15332194

American Psychiatric Association: Diagnostic and Statistical Manual of Mental Disorders, 1st edition. Washington, DC, American Psychiatric Press, 1952

American Psychiatric Association: Diagnostic and Statistical Manual of Mental Disorders, 2nd edition. Washington, DC, American Psychiatric Press, 1968

American Psychiatric Association: Diagnostic and Statistical Manual of Mental
    Disorders, 3rd edition. Washington, DC, American Psychiatric Press, 1980
American Psychiatric Association: Diagnostic and Statistical Manual of Mental
    Disorders, 4th Edition. Washington, DC, American Psychiatric Publishing,
    1994
American Psychiatric Association: Diagnostic and Statistical Manual of Mental
    Disorders, 5th Edition. Arlington, VA, American Psychiatric Publishing, 2013
Anderluh MB, Tchanturia K, Rabe-Hesketh S, et al: Childhood obsessive-
    compulsive personality traits in adult women with eating disorders:
    defining a broader eating disorder phenotype. Am J Psychiatry 160(2):242–
    247, 2003 12562569
Ansell EB, Pinto A, Edelen MO, et al: Structure of Diagnostic and Statistical
    Manual of Mental Disorders, Fourth Ddition criteria for obsessive-
    compulsive personality disorder in patients with binge eating disorder. Can
    J Psychiatry 53(12):863–867, 2008 19087485
Bach B, Anderson JL: Patient-reported ICD-11 personality disorder severity and
    DSM-5 level of personality functioning. J Pers Disord 4:1–19, 2018
    30179575
Bach B, First MB: Application of the ICD-11 classification of personality disorders.
    BMC Psychiatry 18(1):351, 2018 30373564
Bach B, Hutsebaut J: Level of personality functioning scale–brief form 2.0:
    utility in capturing personality problems in psychiatric outpatients and
    incarcerated addicts. J Pers Assess 40(1–2):77–80, 2018 1428984
Bach B, Sellbom M, Kongerslev M, et al: Deriving ICD-11 personality disorder
    domains from DSM-5 traits: initial attempt to harmonize two diagnostic
    systems. Acta Psychiatr Scand 136(1):108–117, 2017 28504853
Bach B, Sellbom M, Skjernov M, et al: ICD-11 and DSM-5 personality trait domains
    capture categorical personality disorders: finding a common ground. Aust N Z
    J Psychiatry 52(5):425–434, 2018 28835108
Butcher JN, Dahlstrom WG, Graham JR, et al: Minnesota Multiphasic Personality
    Inventory, 2nd Edition (MMPI-2). Minneapolis, University of Minnesota
    Press, 1989
Clark LA: Schedule for Nonadaptive and Adaptive Personality (SNAP). Manual
    for Administration, Scoring, and Interpretation. Minneapolis, MN, University
    of Minnesota Press, 1993
Coles ME, Pinto A, Mancebo MC, et al: OCD with comorbid OCPD: a subtype
    of OCD? J Psychiatr Res 42(4):289–296, 2008 17382961
Costa PT Jr, McCrae RR: The five-factor model of personality and its relevance
    to personality disorders. J Pers Disord 6:343–359, 1992
de Reus RJM, Emmelkamp PMG: Obsessive–compulsive personality disorder:
    a review of current empirical findings. Pers Ment Health 6:1–21, 2012
Diedrich A, Voderholzer U: Obsessive-compulsive personality disorder: a
    current review. Curr Psychiatry Rep 17(2):2, 2015 25617042
Ecker W, Kupfer J, Gönner S: Incompleteness as a link between obsessive-
    compulsive personality traits and specific symptom dimensions of
    obsessive-compulsive disorder. Clin Psychol Psychother 21(5):394–402, 2014
    23650140

Farmer RF, Chapman AL: Evaluation of DSM-IV personality disorder criteria as assessed by the structured clinical interview for DSM-IV personality disorders. Compr Psychiatry 43(4):285–300, 2002 12107866

Farnam A, Zamanlu M: Personality disorders: The reformed classification in International Classification of Diseases-11 (ICD-11). Indian J Soc Psychiatry 34:S49–S53, 2018

Fineberg NA, Reghunandanan S, Kolli S, et al: Obsessive-compulsive (anankastic) personality disorder: toward the ICD-11 classification. Br J Psychiatry 36(suppl 1):40–50, 2014 25388611

First MB, Williams JBW, Benjamin LS, et al: User's Guide for the Structured Clinical Interview for DSM-5 Personality Disorders (SCID-5-PD). Arlington, VA, American Psychiatric Association, 2015

First MB, Williams JBW, Benjamin LS, et al: Structured Clinical Interview for DSM-5 Screening Personality Questionnaire (SCID-5-SPQ). Arlington, VA, American Psychiatric Association, 2016

First MB, Skodol AE, Bender DS, et al: Structured Clinical Interview for the DSM-5 Alternative Model for Personality Disorders (SCID-AMPD) Module I: Structured Clinical Interview for the Level of Personality Functioning Scale. Arlington, VA, American Psychiatric Association, 2018a

First MB, Skodol AE, Bender DS, et al: Structured Clinical Interview for the DSM-5 Alternative Model for Personality Disorders (SCID-AMPD) Module III: Structured Clinical Interview for Personality Disorders. Arlington, VA, American Psychiatric Association, 2018b

Fossati A, Beauchaine TP, Grazioli F, et al: Confirmatory factor analyses of DSM-IV Cluster C personality disorder criteria. J Pers Disord 20(2):186–203, 2006 16643123

Furnham A, Milner R, Akhtar R, et al: A review of measures designed to assess DSM-5 personality disorders. Psychology (Irvine) 5:1646–1686, 2014

Grant JE, Mooney ME, Kushner MG: Prevalence, correlates, and comorbidity of DSM-IV obsessive-compulsive personality disorder: results from the National Epidemiologic Survey on Alcohol and Related Conditions. J Psychiatr Res 46(4):469–475, 2012 22257387

Griffin SA, Suzuki T, Lynam DR, et al: Development and examination of the Five-Factor Obsessive-Compulsive Inventory–Short Form. Assessment 25(1):56–68, 2018 27095820

Grilo CM: Factor structure of DSM-IV criteria for obsessive compulsive personality disorder in patients with binge eating disorder. Acta Psychiatr Scand 109(1):64–69, 2004 14674960

Grilo CM, McGlashan TH, Morey LC, et al: Internal consistency, intercriterion overlap and diagnostic efficiency of criteria sets for DSM-IV schizotypal, borderline, avoidant and obsessive-compulsive personality disorders. Acta Psychiatr Scand 104(4):264–272, 2001 11722301

Hertler SC: Understanding obsessive-compulsive personality disorder: reviewing the specificity and sensitivity of DSM-IV diagnostic criteria. Sage Open, July–September 2013. Available at: https://journals.sagepub.com/doi/10.1177/2158244013500675. Accessed April 6, 2019.

Hyler SE: Personality Diagnostic Questionnaire–4 (PDQ-4). New York, New York State Psychiatric Institute, 1994

Hummelen B, Wilberg T, Pedersen G, et al: The quality of the DSM-IV obsessive-compulsive personality disorder construct as a prototype category. J Nerv Ment Dis 196(6):446–455, 2008 18552621

Klein MH, Benjamin LS: The Wisconsin Personality Disorders Inventory–IV. Unpublished test, University of Wisconsin, Madison, WI, 1996 (Available from Dr. MH Klein, Department of Psychiatry, Wisconsin Psychiatric Institute and Clinic, 6001 Research Park Blvd, Madison, WI 53719-1179)

Loranger AW: International Personality Disorder Examination (IPDE). Odessa, FL, Psychological Assessment Resources, 1999

Loranger AW: OMNI Personality Inventory and OMNI-IV Personality Disorder Inventory Manual. Odessa, FL, Psychological Assessment Resources, 2002

Lotfi M, Bach B, Amini M, et al: Structure of DSM-5 and ICD-11 personality domains in Iranian community sample. Pers Ment Health 12(2):155–169, 2018 29392855

Mancebo MC, Eisen JL, Grant JE, et al: Obsessive compulsive personality disorder and obsessive compulsive disorder: clinical characteristics, diagnostic difficulties, and treatment. Ann Clin Psychiatry 17(4):197–204, 2005 16402751

McGlashan TH, Grilo CM, Sanislow CA, et al: Two-year prevalence and stability of individual DSM-IV criteria for schizotypal, borderline, avoidant, and obsessive-compulsive personality disorders: toward a hybrid model of axis II disorders. Am J Psychiatry 162(5):883–889, 2005 15863789

Millon T, Davis R, Millon C: MCMI-III Manual, 2nd Edition. Minneapolis, MN, National Computer Systems, 1997

Mulder RT, Newton-Howes G, Crawford MJ, et al: The central domains of personality pathology in psychiatric patients. J Pers Disord 25(3):364–377, 2011 21699397

Nilsson EW, Gillberg C, Gillberg IC, et al: Ten-year follow-up of adolescent-onset anorexia nervosa: personality disorders. J Am Acad Child Adolesc Psychiatry 38(11):1389–1395, 1999 10560225

O'Connor BP: A search for consensus on the dimensional structure of personality disorders. J Clin Psychol 61(3):323–345, 2005 15468325

Oltmanns JR, Widiger TA: A self-report measure for the ICD-11 dimensional trait model proposal: The Personality Inventory for ICD-11. Psychol Assess 30(2):154–169, 2018 28230410

Phillips KA, McElroy SL: Personality disorders and traits in patients with body dysmorphic disorder. Compr Psychiatry 41(4):229–236, 2000 10929788

Pinto A, Mancebo MC, Eisen JL, et al: The Brown Longitudinal Obsessive Compulsive Study: clinical features and symptoms of the sample at intake. J Clin Psychiatry 67(5):703–711, 2006 16841619

Pinto A, Steinglass JE, Greene AL, et al: Capacity to delay reward differentiates obsessive-compulsive disorder and obsessive-compulsive personality disorder. Biol Psychiatry 75(8):653–659, 2014 24199665

Riddle MA, Maher BS, Wang Y, et al: Obsessive-compulsive personality disorder: evidence for two dimensions. Depress Anxiety 33(2):128–135, 2016 26594839

Sadri SK, McEvoy PM, Pinto A, et al: A psychometric examination of the Pathological Obsessive Compulsive Personality Scale (POPS): initial study in an undergraduate sample. J Pers Assess 1:1–10, 2018 29494778

Samuel DB, Widiger TA: A comparison of obsessive-compulsive personality disorder scales. J Pers Assess 92(3):232–240, 2010 20408023

Samuel DB, Widiger TA: Conscientiousness and obsessive-compulsive personality disorder. Pers Disord 2(3):161–174, 2011 22448765

Samuel DB, Riddell AD, Lynam DR, et al: A five-factor measure of obsessive-compulsive personality traits. J Pers Assess 94(5):456–465, 2012 22519829

Samuels J, Nestadt G, Bienvenu OJ, et al: Personality disorders and normal personality dimensions in obsessive-compulsive disorder. Br J Psychiatry 177:457–462, 2000 11060001

Sanislow CA, Morey LC, Grilo CM, et al: Confirmatory factor analysis of DSM-IV borderline, schizotypal, avoidant and obsessive-compulsive personality disorders: findings from the Collaborative Longitudinal Personality Disorders Study. Acta Psychiatr Scand 105(1):28–36, 2002 12086222

Skodol AE, Gunderson JG, McGlashan TH, et al: Functional impairment in patients with schizotypal, borderline, avoidant, or obsessive-compulsive personality disorder. Am J Psychiatry 159(2):276–283, 2002 11823271

Skodol AE, First MB, Bender DS, Oldham JM: SCID-5-AMPD Structured Clinical Interview for the DSM-5® Alternative Model for Personality Disorders Module II: Structured Clinical Interview for Personality Traits. Arlington, VA, American Psychiatric Association, 2018

Starcevic V, Brakoulias V: New diagnostic perspectives on obsessive-compulsive personality disorder and its links with other conditions. Curr Opin Psychiatry 27(1):62–67, 2014 24257122

Stoeber L, Damian LE: The Clinical Perfectionism Questionnaire: further evidence for two factors capturing perfectionistic strivings and concerns. Pers Individ Dif 61–62:38–42, 2014

Summerfeldt LJ: Understanding and treating incompleteness in obsessive-compulsive disorder. J Clin Psychol 60(11):1155–1168, 2004 15389620

Summerfeldt LJ, Antony MM, Swinson RP: Incompleteness: a link between perfectionistic traits and OCD. Presented at the Association for the Advancement of Behavior Therapy meeting, New Orleans, LA, 2000

Tyrer P, Crawford M, Mulder R, et al: The rationale for the reclassification of personality disorder in the 11th revision of the International Classification of Diseases (ICD-11). Pers Ment Health 5:246–259, 2011

Tyrer P, Reed GM, Crawford MJ: Classification, assessment, prevalence, and effect of personality disorder. Lancet 385(9969):717–726, 2015 25706217

Veale D, Boocock A, Gournay K, et al: Body dysmorphic disorder: a survey of fifty cases. Br J Psychiatry 169(2):196–201, 1996 8871796

Widiger TA, Boyd S: Personality disorders assessment instruments, in Oxford Handbook of Personality Assessment. Edited by Butcher JN. New York, Oxford University Press, 2009, pp 336–363

Widiger TA, Mullins-Sweatt SN: Clinical utility of a dimensional model of personality disorder. Prof Psychol Res Pr 41:488, 2010

Widiger TA, Simonsen E: Alternative dimensional models of personality disorder: finding a common ground. J Pers Disord 19(2):110–130, 2005 15899712

Widiger TA, Mangine S, Corbitt EM: Personality Disorder Interview–IV: A Semi-structured Interview for the Assessment of Personality Disorders. Professional Manual. Odessa, FL, Psychological Assessment Resources, 1995

Widiger TA, Trull TJ, Clarkin JF, et al: A description of the DSM-IV personality disorders with the five-factor model of personality, in Personality Disorders and the Five-Factor Model of Personality, 2nd Edition. Edited by Costa PT Jr, Widiger TA. Washington, DC, American Psychological Association, 2002, pp 89–99

World Health Organization: The ICD-10 Classification of Mental and Behavioural Disorders: Clinical Descriptions and Diagnostic Guidelines. Geneva, World Health Organization, 1992

World Health Organization: Mental, behavioural or neurodevelomental disorders, in International Classification of Diseases-11 for Mortality and Morbidity Statistics. Geneva, World Health Organization, 2019

Zanarini MC, Frankenburg FR, Sickel AE, et al: The Diagnostic Interview for DSM-IV Personality Disorders (DIPD-IV). Belmont, MA, McLean Hospital, 1996

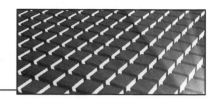

CHAPTER 3

OCPD AND ITS RELATIONSHIP TO OBSESSIVE-COMPULSIVE AND HOARDING DISORDERS

Michael G. Wheaton, Ph.D.
Anthony Pinto, Ph.D.

CASE VIGNETTES

Case 1

Monica, a 28-year-old married female, presented for treatment of primary obsessive-compulsive disorder (OCD). Her OCD symptoms included intrusive thoughts about contamination (obsessions) as well as repetitive washing behaviors (compulsions). For example, Monica was

49

preoccupied with the idea that her countertops or floor might be covered in harmful bacteria, such as salmonella, and she would spend about an hour per day wiping down her counters and floors with disinfectant wipes. She also washed her hands excessively and had an extensive ritual for household chores such as doing the laundry or putting away groceries. These symptoms fit with the prototypical presentations of OCD, and Monica's treatment included deliberate practices at confronting contamination-provoking stimuli (exposures) and refraining from ritualistic washing (response prevention). However, in addition to these OCD symptoms, Monica presented with symptoms of obsessive-compulsive personality disorder (OCPD), including perfectionism, preoccupation with orderliness and detail, interpersonal rigidity, and difficulty delegating tasks. Some of these symptoms related directly to her OCD symptoms. For example, she described needing to clean until things were "perfectly" cleaned, paying particular attention to tiny flecks or crumbs that might have landed on the floor, and having rigid standards for cleaning (e.g., requiring her husband to use disinfecting wipes when he spilled breakfast cereal on the floor) and being interpersonally controlling (e.g., not allowing her husband to do the laundry because he wouldn't do it "right").

In addition, some of the features of Monica's OCPD manifested independently of her OCD symptoms. For example, she frequently avoided making decisions out of fear that she might make the wrong choice (e.g., she procrastinated on buying a new dishwasher for months because she needed to find the "perfect" one), and she was frequently late in submitting assignments required for the classes she was taking in pursuit of a graduate degree. Importantly, although she recognized that her fears of contracting an illness from household contaminants were excessive and unreasonable, Monica had less insight into the maladaptive nature of her personality traits and associated behaviors. These tendencies also impacted her ability to successfully complete the OCD treatment she had initially sought because she was often late for sessions due to getting "stuck" seeking perfection at tasks and also avoided doing therapy homework when she felt she did not have enough time to do it "perfectly."

Case 2

Erik, a 45-year-old married white male, presented for treatment with a commonly observed constellation of OCPD symptoms: maladaptive perfectionism; interpersonal rigidity; rigidly held morals, ethics, and values; and the tendency to attempt to exert control over the environment in service of rigid standards for conduct and behavior. In addition, Erik's symptoms manifested with a particular focus on material objects. Erik was preoccupied by the idea that excessive consumption of material goods was causing irreparable harm to the environment. As a result, Erik adopted an extremely rigid set of rules to reduce his own (and his family's) consumption of nonbiodegradable items and endeavored to maximally reuse and recycle everything they acquired. For example, when going to pick up food at a takeout restaurant, he would take his own food containers so that he would not be given plastic food containers or utensils. He would also sort through the trash in his apartment building to remove items that could have been recycled rather than thrown out and occasionally confronted his neighbors for being "wasteful." He also collected items that he believed could be repurposed, such as plastic tubing and plastic containers. These items began to clutter his apartment and caused interpersonal conflict with his wife, who did not like that their home was being used to store so many items that were never used. Erik was also interpersonally controlling of his possessions, forbidding his family members from touching them or throwing them out without his permission. He presented for treatment hoping to reduce the marital conflict he and his wife were experiencing. He denied, however, that his difficulty with saving possessions and his tendency to be rigid or controlling were problematic in themselves. Rather, he desired to find a way to convince his spouse to "get off his back" and see that his behaviors were in fact proper and appropriate.

The notion that OCPD and OCD are linked traces back more than 100 years, predating the development of the current diagnostic system. For example, Janet (1904) proposed that OCD was preceded by a period he described as a *psychasthenic state*, which included perfectionism, indecisiveness, and emotional detachment. Similarly, Freud linked the development of OCD to the *anal character*, which involved obstinacy, excessive orderliness, and undue miserliness ((Freud 1908/1959)). As diagnostic systems have been refined over time, the link between OCD and OCPD has endured. Subsequent refinements to the diagnostic system separated hoarding symptoms to identify an independent disorder, hoarding disorder (HD), which has also been linked to OCPD. These three conditions—OCPD, OCD, and HD—clearly share some associations, yet their relationship has been frequently misunderstood. In this chapter, we aim to shed light on the similarities and differences among these disorders, as well as to characterize the nature of their co-occurrence. Importantly, we focus on reviewing relationships among these conditions as they are currently classified according to the fifth edition of the *Diagnostic and Statistical Manual of Mental Disorders* (DSM-5; American Psychiatric Association 2013). We reserve consideration of dimensional approaches to OCPD to our section on future research presented at the end of the chapter.

The case vignettes described above illustrate a small cross-section of the often complicated relationships between OCPD and OCD or between OCPD and hoarding symptoms. In the first case, Monica suffers from both OCPD and OCD, and although she presented for treatment for OCD, her OCPD appears to warrant clinical attention as well, insofar as it appears to be complicating her OCD treatment. In the second case, Erik presented for treatment of primary OCPD, but saving excessive items in his home resulted in clutter, a symptom of HD; however, because Erik felt no sentimental attachment to his possessions, and the degree of clutter in his home was not substantial enough to cause the loss of functionality of the living space, it appears that his hoarding symptoms were at a subthreshold level and would not meet full diagnostic criteria for HD. In this chapter, we aim to describe the complicated relationship between these conditions as illustrated in these two cases. First, we focus on the relationship between OCPD and OCD, followed by that between OCPD and HD.

OCPD AND OBSESSIVE-COMPULSIVE DISORDER

Symptoms, Core Components, and Differential Diagnosis

OCD is a chronic condition estimated to affect up to 2% of the population (Ruscio et al. 2010). OCD can be disabling when severe and is estimated to be an important cause of illness-related disability around the world (Murray et al. 1996). OCD is characterized by intrusive and unwanted thoughts, images, or urges that provoke distress (obsessions) and/or repetitive behaviors or mental acts that aim to relieve distress or prevent feared consequences (compulsions) (American Psychiatric Association 2013).

The association between OCPD and OCD traces back many years. Early psychoanalysts often described the features of both OCD and OCPD as obsessive-compulsive neurosis (Angyal 1965). Indeed, there is some overlap in terms of the symptoms of both conditions at the topographical level (i.e., the form of symptoms). For example, excessive list making can be a compulsive behavior in individuals with either OCPD or OCD. In OCPD, writing extensive lists often results from a preoccupation with details and a drive for completion. List making is also seen as a compulsive behavior in OCD and is included on the symptom checklist that accompanies the most widely used measure of OCD severity, the Yale-Brown Obsessive Compulsive Scale (Y-BOCS; Goodman et al. 1989). However, as we have described elsewhere (Pinto et al. 2018; Wheaton and Pinto 2017), the symptoms of OCD and OCPD appear to spring from distinct motivations when analyzed on a functional level.

In OCD, symptoms are time consuming, intrusive, and distressing (American Psychiatric Association 2013). In addition, the great majority of OCD patients have sufficient insight to recognize that their symptoms are excessive and irrational (American Psychiatric Association

2013). Thus, OCD symptoms are typically considered to be *ego-dystonic* because they do not align with the individual's sense of self and values (i.e., the symptoms are upsetting and unwanted). In comparison, the symptomatic traits and behaviors associated with OCPD are usually thought to be ego-syntonic because the individual experiences them as being appropriate and proper (in line with his or her sense of self). Although distress is experienced in individuals with both conditions, in OCD the distress is typically experienced as a result of the symptoms themselves (i.e., the presence of upsetting thoughts, images, or urges), whereas in OCPD the distress often comes secondary to the conflict and discrepancy between the OCPD traits and the external world. For example, distress in OCPD can result from the discrepancy between ideals of perfection and actual performance that does not live up to those standards. Similarly, distress and interpersonal conflict can result from attempting to impose rigid rules for conduct on other people (i.e., attempts to control others). In line with this proposition, although both OCD and OCPD often involve time-consuming and methodical behaviors (e.g., writing and rewriting work, organizing and arranging belongings, making lists), they can be differentiated by the presence of obsessions in OCD (Pinto et al. 2014). Therefore, current consensus conceptualizes OCD and OCPD as distinct diagnostic entities (Pinto et al. 2018).

Although distinct, OCD and OCPD may share some core contributing features. Of these, perfectionism may be the most salient. Maladaptive perfectionism (defined by Frost et al. [1990] as the tendency to set and pursue unrealistically high standards and to employ overly critical self-evaluations) is considered to be at the core of the OCPD construct. Yet perfectionism has also been thought of as a contributing factor to OCD symptoms. For example, in studying the cognitive factors involved in OCD, the Obsessive Compulsive Cognitions Working Group (1997) included a measure of perfectionism as a belief domain—along with responsibility, overestimation of threat, importance of thoughts, control of thoughts, and intolerance of uncertainty—thought to be central to the etiology and maintenance of OCD. Indeed, patients with OCD demonstrate elevated levels of perfectionism compared with healthy controls (Antony et al. 1998a, 1998b). The relationship between perfectionism and OCD symptoms also extends to nonclinical populations, for whom measures of perfectionism are positively correlated with measures of obsessive-compulsive symptoms (Frost et al. 1994; Rhéaume et al. 1995).

These findings suggest that excessive perfectionism is not specific to OCPD, a claim that is in line with the notion that perfectionism represents a transdiagnostic phenomenon (Egan et al. 2011), having also been linked to depression (Rice and Aldea 2006), eating disorders (Fairburn et al. 2003), and other personality disorders (Stoeber 2014). Therefore, perfectionism may be central to the psychopathology of OCD, OCPD, and other mental illnesses.

Family History Linkage

Some data hint at a familial link between OCPD and OCD, although the search for a common genetic vulnerability factor has not yet resulted in conclusive results. Several early reports found increased rates of OCPD traits in the parents of children with OCD (Lenane et al. 1990; Swedo et al. 1989), although these reports did not use specifically validated measures of OCPD traits. Subsequently, Samuels et al. (2000) also reported elevated OCPD frequency in first-degree relatives of OCD probands compared with relatives of control probands (11.5% vs. 5.8%, respectively) using the Structured Interview for DSM-III-R Personality (SIDP-R; Pfohl et al. 1989). Calvo et al. (2009) reported on OCPD traits in parents of children with OCD and healthy controls, finding that perfectionism, as well as hoarding and preoccupation with details, occurred significantly more frequently in parents of children with OCD. In addition, certain OCD symptoms (counting, ordering, and cleaning compulsions) in children with OCD were associated with greater likelihood of parental perfectionism and rigidity. However, to date the specific genes that may confer a shared vulnerability to both OCPD and OCD have yet to be identified. It remains unknown whether a third variable, such as neuroticism, may explain the familial association between OCPD and OCD.

Courses of OCD and OCPD

As mentioned previously, early views suggested that certain OCPD traits (e.g., rigidity, miserliness) were expressed prior to the development of OCD. However, relatively little research has tracked the longitudinal association between OCPD and OCD to determine whether in fact people do "convert" from OCPD to OCD. A study of adults found childhood OCPD traits to be linked to adult diagnosis of OCD, although the study used a retrospective design (Pinto et al. 2015). The authors administered the Childhood Retrospective Perfectionism Questionnaire (CHIRP; Southgate et al. 2008)—a validated measure of perfectionism, inflexibility, and drive for order—to samples of adults with OCD without OCPD ($n=28$), OCPD without OCD ($n=27$), or both OCD and OCPD ($n=28$) and to healthy control subjects ($n=28$). They reported that subjects with OCD (without OCPD) had higher rates of inflexibility and drive for order compared with healthy control subjects, suggesting that these traits may presage the development of OCD, independent of OCPD. In addition, after controlling for OCPD diagnosis, childhood obsessive-compulsive personality traits were associated with particular OCD presentations (contamination/washing, doubting/checking, and symmetry/ordering symptoms) (Pinto et al. 2015). Similarly, in a subsequent study of children with OCD, Park et al. (2016) reported that obsessive-compulsive personality traits in youth (using the CHIRP) were associated with concurrent checking, symmetry, and contamination OCD symptom dimensions. These data hint that childhood OCPD traits may indeed be linked to concurrent or subsequent OCD (at least in some forms), although longitudinal research is needed.

In addition, two investigations have studied individuals who had OCD in childhood to assess for OCPD in adulthood. In the first, Thomsen and Mikkelsen (1993) compared children hospitalized for OCD with those hospitalized for a different psychiatric disorder. They reported that both groups had similar rates of personality disorders in general and OCPD in particular. However, OCPD was more common in subjects whose OCD persisted into adulthood compared with the patients who no longer had OCD at follow-up (Thomsen and Mikkelsen 1993). The second study had a similar design but found that OCPD did not differentiate between individuals with persistent OCD versus those whose OCD remitted (Swedo et al. 1989). However, these studies both predated the current diagnostic system for OCPD and OCD codified in DSM-IV (American Psychiatric Association 2000).

Two more recent studies (using DSM-IV criteria) examined longitudinal associations between the disorders but found conflicting results. Analyzing data from the Collaborative Longitudinal Personality Disorders Study (Gunderson et al. 2000), Shea et al. (2004) did not find a clear association between the course of OCD and the course of OCPD. However, in the Brown Longitudinal Obsessive Compulsive Study (Pinto et al. 2006), among patients with OCD, the presence of comorbid OCPD was associated with a poorer course of OCD. Specifically, patients with OCD and comorbid OCPD at intake were only half as likely to remit from OCD after 2 years relative to those without comorbid OCPD at intake (Eisen et al. 2006). On the basis of the mixed results reviewed here, the longitudinal associations between OCPD and OCD remain somewhat unclear and represent an important area for future research.

Comorbidity and Correlates

Although they are best conceptualized as distinct diagnostic entities (as illustrated in Figure 3–1), OCD and OCPD can and do co-occur. Studies of the comorbidity rates between OCD and OCPD have found high rates of OCPD in patients with OCD, ranging from 23% to 32% (Albert et al. 2004; Pinto et al. 2006; Samuels et al. 2000). Data from treatment trials suggest that this rate may be even higher in treatment-seeking samples (47.3%; Starcevic et al. 2013). As mentioned previously, OCD is known as a heterogeneous condition with multiple symptom dimensions. OCPD has shown a specific relationship with particular forms of

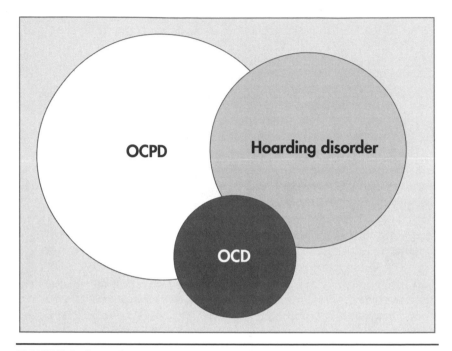

FIGURE 3–1.   Theoretical model of the overlap between obsessive-compulsive personality disorder (OCPD), obsessive-compulsive disorder (OCD), and hoarding disorder.

Note.   OCD is estimated to occur in approximately 2% of the population, hoarding disorder in about 5%, and OCPD in up to 8%.

OCD symptoms. For example, in a study involving a large sample of patients with OCD (*N*=238), Coles et al. (2008) reported that those patients with comorbid OCPD (*n*=65) had higher rates of symmetry and hoarding obsessions and of cleaning, ordering, repeating, and hoarding compulsions. Other studies have linked comorbid OCPD to forms of OCD motivated by incompleteness (Summerfeldt 2004), which refers to an inner sense of imperfection or the feeling that things are "not just right." Symptoms in this dimension can also include the need for symmetry and order coupled with arranging compulsions, as well as the need to repeat activities until done just so. Broader than formal diagnosis of OCPD, so-called "not just right" experiences have been linked to OCPD traits evaluated dimensionally (Ecker et al. 2014).

Much of the work on the relationship between OCD and OCPD has focused on studying patients with a primary diagnosis of OCD, and therefore much less is known about how frequently patients with OCPD also have OCD. However, it would seem that OCD would actually be relatively uncommon among patients with OCPD, based on the differing prevalence estimates for the two disorders (1.2% for OCD and up to 7.9% for OCPD; American Psychiatric Association 2013). As illustrated in Figure 3–1, OCD occurs in a minority of individuals with OCPD. Empirical studies are in line with this notion: in the Collaborative Longitudinal Personality Disorders Study sample, 20.9% of individuals meeting criteria for OCPD were also diagnosed with OCD (McGlashan et al. 2000). Because data on OCPD samples are so limited, further study is necessary.

Treatment Implications

Data are somewhat mixed on the treatment implications of the combined presentation of OCPD and OCD. Given that little research has focused on treatment of OCPD as a primary treatment target (see Chapter 11, "Impact of Personality Disorders on Parenting," and Chapter 12, "Positive Aspects of OCPD," for details), most of the existing research on this combined presentation has focused on the effects of treating OCD when OCPD is comorbid. Current treatment guidelines of the American Psychiatric Association (Koran and Simpson 2013) recommend that OCD be treated with either serotonin reuptake inhibitor (SRI) medications or cognitive-behavioral therapy (CBT), particularly that consisting of exposure with response prevention (EX/RP). These first-line treatments allow many, if not most, OCD patients to benefit. However, some data suggest that comorbid OCPD may make these treatments less effective, as described here.

In terms of SRI medication, fairly few trials have examined the effect of comorbid OCPD on pharmacotherapy outcomes for OCD. In one trial of clomipramine and fluvoxamine, Cavedini et al. (1997) compared outcomes of 9 patients with OCD and OCPD and 29 patients with OCD without OCPD and found that those with co-occurring OCPD had significantly less improvement in their OCD symptoms. However, other trials have found that comorbid OCPD was not predictive of worse outcomes with medication (Baer et al. 1990). Therefore, more research is needed in this area.

In terms of psychotherapy for OCD, multiple variants of CBT have been found to be effective (Skapinakis et al. 2016), including cognitive therapy and behaviorally focused EX/RP. Whereas cognitive therapy involves rationally restructuring maladaptive OCD-related beliefs and cognitions, EX/RP involves repeated confrontations with feared stimuli and situations (exposures) as well as practice refraining from compulsive rituals (response prevention). Unfortunately, although substantial research has examined the efficacy of CBT variants at reducing OCD symptoms, relatively few studies have explored the effects of comorbid OCPD on CBT outcomes, and the data that do exist are somewhat mixed. In one well-controlled trial of manualized EX/RP, Pinto et al. (2011) found that comorbid OCPD was linked to poorer OCD treatment outcomes. In contrast, in a study of patients receiving more cognitively based CBT (using cognitive restructuring and behavioral experiments to change underlying beliefs), Gordon et al. (2016) reported that patients with OCD and OCPD actually had *better* outcomes compared with patients without comorbid OCPD. These opposite findings merit reflection and consideration. One possibility, as proposed by Gordon et al. (2016), is that comorbid OCPD may have more negative impact in a behaviorally based treatment (EX/RP) than in cognitively based CBT. Therefore, the effect of OCPD may depend on the specific variant of CBT employed to treat OCD.

An alternative possibility is that studying the categorical presence versus absence of OCPD may not be the optimal way to predict treatment outcomes because doing so introduces heterogeneity of symptom presentations that may produce inconsistent results across samples. Coding OCPD as present versus absent ignores the fact that the polythetic diagnostic criteria of OCPD mean that multiple constellations of symptoms can result in the diagnosis of OCPD, whereas some individuals may endorse some of the most important OCPD symptoms but fail to meet official diagnostic criteria because they fall just short of the number needed for diagnosis. Some researchers (e.g., Widiger and Sanderson 1995) have criticized the categorical system and instead suggested that dimensional measures of personality pathology may be better (Widiger 2007). Therefore, examining personality trait dimensions may be a more optimal strategy for exploring how aspects of the OCPD construct relate to the effectiveness of CBT for OCD (Starcevic and Brakoulias 2014).

As discussed earlier in the section on OCPD and OCD symptoms, core components, and differential diagnosis, among the features thought to be at the core of the OCPD construct, maladaptive perfectionism is one of the most stable and prevalent OCPD features (McGlashan et al. 2005). Importantly, perfectionism has been studied as a transdiagnostic phenomenon (Egan et al. 2011) that can lead to significant distress and functional impairment independently and through other psychological disorders and has been linked to depression (Blatt et al. 1995, 1998; Rice and Aldea 2006), suicidality (O'Connor 2007), and eating disorders (Egan et al. 2011). Therefore, perfectionism may have implications for OCD treatment, and indeed it seems most linked to OCD treatment outcomes. In their study of outpatients receiving EX/RP, Pinto et al. (2011) examined the impact of individual OCPD symptoms and found that only perfectionism was linked with poor OCD outcomes, whereas the other OCPD symptoms (e.g., preoccupation with details, miserliness, hypermorality) were not. In line with this finding, Kyrios et al. (2015)

examined predictors of outcomes among 79 patients receiving outpatient CBT (which included both cognitive therapy and EX/RP) and reported that baseline scores on the Perfectionism/Need for Certainty subscale of the Obsessive Belief Questionnaire (OBQ; Obsessive Compulsive Cognitions Working Group 2005) predicted treatment outcomes, such that greater perfectionism or intolerance of uncertainty was associated with higher posttreatment scores, accounting for baseline severity. Although these data are somewhat limited because this measure combines perfectionism with another construct (intolerance of uncertainty), they are in line with the notion that more perfectionistic OCD patients may fare worse in CBT.

Pinto et al. (2011) outlined four ways in which perfectionism may interfere with CBT for OCD: 1) when patients' attempts to do the treatment "perfectly" end up backfiring, 2) when patients avoid or do not fully adhere to assigned between-session CBT tasks because of fear of not doing the tasks correctly, 3) when patients take a narrow view of exposures and do not generalize to new situations, and 4) when patients give up on trying in treatment if they believe they are not making perfect progress. Notably, in the Gordon et al. (2016) study that found OCPD to be linked to better CBT outcomes, the authors did not specifically investigate the impact of perfectionism in particular. Therefore, more research is needed to explore the relationship between perfectionism and OCD treatment outcomes.

Some data also suggest that perfectionism improves when CBT for OCD is successful. For example, multiple clinical trials of CBT for OCD have reported that scores on the OBQ (including the Perfectionism/Certainty subscale) are reduced from baseline to posttreatment (Pinto et al. 2017). Kyrios et al. (2015) extended these results by examining whether improved OBQ subscale scores predict degree of improvement in OCD symptoms. They reported that reduced Perfectionism/Certainty scores significantly accounted for improvement in OCD symptoms. These results suggest that improving perfectionism may significantly account for OCD improvement. Improving perfectionism might therefore be an important mediator of OCD improvement, and reducing perfectionism could therefore be an important target in OCD treatment. Importantly, CBT treatment interventions have been specifically developed to target perfectionism (Egan et al. 2011, 2013), and future research could investigate the possibility that incorporating these interventions might improve treatment for patients with co-occurring OCD and OCPD with high levels of perfectionism.

OCPD AND HOARDING DISORDER

Symptoms, Core Components, and Differential Diagnosis

As described elsewhere in this volume, one of the current diagnostic symptoms for OCPD, as defined in DSM-5 (American Psychiatric Association 2013), is difficulty discarding worn-out or useless items. This item overlaps considerably with the core element of hoarding—persistent difficulty discarding or parting with possessions, regardless of their actual value (American Psychiatric Association 2013). This overlap in symptoms can make it difficult for clinicians to differentiate between these two conditions and merits special reflection. To begin with, the relationship between hoarding and OCD and OCPD has been the subject of much debate and confusion tracing back many decades. For example, Freud (1959) theorized that hoarding behavior was part of the anal triad of orderliness, parsimony, and obstinacy and that these factors were often a precursor to OCD. Speculation regarding the link between OCD, OCPD, and hoarding has continued for more than a century. In previous DSM editions, difficulty discarding possessions served as an overlapping link between OCPD and OCD. For instance, according to DSM-IV, difficulty discarding worthless or worn-out items should be seen as a diagnostic criterion for OCPD, but when saving behavior is extreme, a diagnosis of OCD was recommended (American Psychiatric Association 2000). As substantial theoretical and empirical research accumulated (Mataix-Cols et al. 2010; Wheaton et al. 2011), the DSM-5 committee elected to separate hoarding from OCD by creating an independent HD category.

According to DSM-5 (American Psychiatric Association 2013), the diagnostic criteria for HD are as follows:

1. Persistent difficulty discarding or parting with possessions, regardless of their actual value.
2. This difficulty is due to a perceived need to save the items and to distress associated with discarding them.
3. Saving possessions results in accumulation of significant clutter that impairs function of living space.
4. Clinically significant distress or impairment in social, occupational, or other functioning (including a safe living environment).
5. The problem is not attributable to another medical condition or mental disorder.

HD appears to be surprisingly common. DSM-5 estimates a 2%–6% lifetime prevalence rate for HD in the United States (American Psychiatric Association 2013).

HD and OCPD can be challenging to differentiate, but several features may help in differentiating them. First, whereas the accumulated possessions of individuals with OCPD are frequently orderly and neat, those of individuals with HD are typically disorganized and stored without a systematic organization system. Second, individuals with HD frequently engage in excessive acquisition of unnecessary items (excessive acquisition is included as a DSM-5 specifier for HD). These excessive acquisition behaviors may be less common in individuals with OCPD, who are typically reserved about spending money (i.e., miserly). Indeed, findings from one study suggest that in a monetary incentive reward task, individuals with OCPD may show an abnormally strong ability to delay rewards (as compared with both individuals with OCD and healthy controls) (Pinto et al. 2014), which would seem to differentiate individuals with OCPD from those with HD, whose inability to deny immediate gratification results in excessive acquisition. Third, individuals with OCPD and HD might be differentiated on the basis of their reasons for saving possessions. Substantial previous work has investigated the reasons why individuals with HD have difficulty parting with possessions (Steketee et al. 2003). Although there is quite a lot of heterogeneity, common reasons for saving items in HD include feeling sentimentally attached to possessions, which has been termed *hypersentimentality* (e.g., feeling that throwing away a possession causes it "emotional" harm), as well as concerns that items are needed because of concerns about memory (e.g., believing that parting with a possession will result in a loss of an ability to remember an important experience). Although much less research has investigated reasons for saving items in OCPD, these common HD reasons for saving may not always be observed in OCPD, where the difficulty discarding old or worn-out items may function to "maximize" their use (i.e., a manifestation of perfectionism). For instance, an individual with OCPD may hold on to a pile of magazines, newspapers, or other reading material because he or she has not read them entirely and therefore has not derived full benefit from them.

Finally (and perhaps most obviously), the total amount of possessions and the extent of clutter may help to differentiate the conditions because in HD the clutter must be substantial enough to disrupt the usability of some living space (e.g., a living room so cluttered that no one can sit on the chairs and couch or a bedroom in which the bed is covered with material such that it cannot be slept in). Thus, clutter in HD is substantial enough to impair basic activities (e.g., moving through the house, completing activities such as cooking and cleaning) or represents a significant hazard (e.g., lack of access to emergency exits, fire or pest hazards). Saving of possessions in uncomplicated OCPD would not be expected to result in such extreme levels of clutter (and were such levels of clutter to be observed, likely both HD and OCPD should be diagnosed). It should be noted, however, that the inability to discard worn-out or useless items is considered to be one of the least central of all the OCPD diagnostic criteria to the overall OCPD construct. For example, a factor analysis of OCPD symptoms found that the symptom of discarding worthless or worn-out items did not load on the OCPD factor and did not discriminate between OCPD and other Cluster C personality disorders (Fossati et al. 2006). It has therefore been recommended that this item be dropped as an OCPD criterion (Diedrich and Voderholzer 2015). However, as discussed in the next subsection, the association between OCPD and HD may remain substantial even without this diagnostic symptom overlap.

Comorbidity and Correlates

It is difficult to evaluate the rate of comorbid HD in individuals with OCPD because previous large-scale epidemiological (Grant et al. 2012) and longitudinal (McGlashan et al. 2005) studies of OCPD have not reported on rates of this comorbidity. A major challenge to this work, of course, is that formal diagnostic criteria for HD were codified only relatively recently with the publication of DSM-5 (American Psychiatric Association 2013). Therefore, future work in this area is clearly necessary.

Slightly more data exist from studies focused on individuals with HD; these studies have generally reported that a substantial minority of individuals with HD met criteria for comorbid OCPD. For example, Frost et al. (2011) characterized comorbidity patterns in a sample of 217 individuals with primary HD as well as 96 comparison subjects diagnosed with OCD without HD. They reported that 29.5% of the HD participants had comorbid OCPD, a rate significantly higher than that among the OCD participants, 16.7% of whom had comorbid OCPD. However, recognizing the potential for diagnostic "double counting" of discarding difficulty, the authors calculated how many subjects in the sample would meet criteria for OCPD after excluding hoarding possessions as an OCPD criterion. With this "stricter" definition of OCPD, the two groups did not significantly differ, in that 18.8% of the HD group and 14.6% of the OCD group met reduced OCPD criteria. This study suggests that some of the comorbidity between OCPD and HD is driven by overlap in saving items, yet this hoarding criterion did not fully account for the relationship between the two disorders: even when hoarding was removed as a criterion, OCPD was the most common comorbid personality disorder with HD, occurring more than twice as often as avoidant personality disorder, which was the next most common personality disorder seen in HD participants (8.8%). This result is in line with a previous study, albeit with a smaller sample size: Landau et al. (2011) found that 50% of 24 individuals with HD also had OCPD, and the rate was 33.3% even when hoarding was excluded as an OCPD criterion. In particular, hoarding symptoms have been linked to symptoms of perfectionism (Frost and Gross 1993), again in line with the notion that perfectionism may be a transdiagnostic factor that might contribute to OCPD, OCD, and HD. The potential overlap between OCPD and HD is also demonstrated in Figure 3–1.

Treatment Implications

Substantially less research has examined treatments for HD than for OCD. Past research considering hoarding symptoms within the context of OCD found that OCD patients with hoarding problems evidence worse treatment outcomes compared with patients with other OCD symptoms (Bloch et al. 2014). This spurred researchers to investigate hoarding-specific treatment options. Of these, CBT for HD has been the most systematically studied, with research supporting the use of CBT to reduce HD symptoms when delivered in both individual (Steketee et al. 2010) and group (Gilliam et al. 2011) formats. CBT for HD is a multicomponent treatment that begins with a detailed assessment of the hoarding symptoms and development of an individualized case conceptualization of contributing factors. Treatment includes skills training in categorizing, organizing, and problem solving, as well as practice with sorting, decision making, and discarding both in session and as homework. In addition, clinicians can incorporate techniques from motivational interviewing to address ambivalence and low insight. Many individuals benefit from this treatment, with estimates of response rates suggesting that 70%–80% of patients are much or very much improved after 9–12 months of treatment. These improvements were largely maintained at 1-year follow-up (Steketee et al. 2010).

Unfortunately, to date no study has formally evaluated the effect of comorbid OCPD on the effectiveness of CBT for HD. However, a study that examined predictors of outcomes in a sample of 37 individuals receiving 26 sessions of individual CBT for HD reported that perfectionism was significantly associated with worse treatment outcomes (Muroff et al. 2014). Specifically, individuals with higher levels of perfectionism had greater posttreatment HD severity, even after accounting for baseline severity. Although these results require replication, they align with some previous work on OCD in suggesting that maladaptive perfectionism may interfere with treatment. To the extent that perfectionism represents a core OCPD feature, these data suggest that OCPD may also be a complicating factor in treating HD.

FUTURE DIRECTIONS FOR RESEARCH

As reviewed in this chapter and illustrated in the case vignettes, the relationships between OCPD, OCD, and HD are complicated and full of nuance. In some instances, such as in Monica's case, OCD and OCPD can co-occur. In these cases, treating one condition (OCD in the case of Monica) can be made more difficult by the comorbid condition (OCPD). In Erik's case, symptoms of hoarding (accumulation of clutter) related directly to core features of OCPD (rigid rules, hypermorality, perfectionism, and difficulty delegating). Together, these cases illustrate the need for treating clinicians to carefully evaluate differential diagnosis, including examining the function of behaviors and whether they are ego-syntonic or ego-dystonic, and to assess for the presence of OCPD traits in their patients with OCD and HD. These cases illustrate the potential for OCPD traits to present challenges in treatment, including with pharmacotherapy or psychotherapy. Importantly, although OCD and HD have been historically linked to OCPD for many decades, important aspects of these associations and how best to treat these comorbid presentations remain understudied.

It is noteworthy that we have focused on reviewing the research base on OCPD, OCD, and HD as they are currently conceptualized and diagnosed. At the same time, however, a major research endeavor is currently evaluating a reconceptualization of personality disorders to be more dimensional as opposed to categorical. This area of research offers great promise to clarify and better understand the relationships between OCPD and OCD and between OCPD and HD. Focusing on particular OCPD trait dimensions (e.g., maladaptive perfectionism, rigidity) may allow researchers to avoid some of the issues of diagnostic overlap described in this chapter (i.e., by removing "difficulty discarding items" as a symptom of OCPD). Although this work is in its nascent stages, it appears that maladaptive perfectionism represents a core OCPD trait dimension that has great importance for understanding the relationship between OCPD, OCD, and HD. This is especially true to the extent that maladaptive perfectionism can be specifically targeted in treatment, which may allow for more successful treatments for patients with OCD or HD who also experience OCPD. The upcoming years of research in this area offer great promise to improve the current understanding of these conditions and ways to treat them.

TAKE-HOME POINTS

- Historically, OCPD has been linked to both OCD and HD.
- Although OCPD, OCD, and HD share some associated features, they represent distinct diagnostic categories.
- Maladaptive perfectionism may be a feature shared by all three conditions.
- Comorbidity among OCPD, OCD, and HD is relatively common and may have implications for treatment.

REFERENCES

Albert U, Maina G, Forner F, et al: DSM-IV obsessive-compulsive personality disorder: prevalence in patients with anxiety disorders and in healthy comparison subjects. Compr Psychiatry 45(5):325–332, 2004 15332194

American Psychiatric Association: Diagnostic and Statistical Manual of Mental Disorders, 4th Edition, Text Revision. Washington, DC, American Psychiatric Association, 2000

American Psychiatric Association: Diagnostic and Statistical Manual of Mental Disorders, 5th Edition. Arlington, VA, American Psychiatric Publishing, 2013

Angyal A: Neurosis and Treatment: A Holistic Theory. New York, Wiley, 1965

Antony MM, Downie F, Swinson RP: Diagnostic issues and epidemiology in obsessive-compulsive disorder, in Obsessive-Compulsive Disorder: Theory, Research, and Treatment. New York, Guilford, 1998a, pp 3–32

Antony MM, Purdon CL, Huta V, et al: Dimensions of perfectionism across the anxiety disorders. Behav Res Ther 36(12):1143–1154, 1998b 9745799

Baer L, Jenike MA, Ricciardi JN 2nd, et al: Standardized assessment of personality disorders in obsessive-compulsive disorder. Arch Gen Psychiatry 47(9):826–830, 1990 2393341

Blatt SJ, Quinlan DM, Pilkonis PA, et al: Impact of perfectionism and need for approval on the brief treatment of depression: the National Institute of Mental Health Treatment of Depression Collaborative Research Program revisited. J Consult Clin Psychol 63(1):125–132, 1995 7896977

Blatt SJ, Zuroff DC, Bondi CM, et al: When and how perfectionism impedes the brief treatment of depression: further analyses of the National Institute of Mental Health Treatment of Depression Collaborative Research Program. J Consult Clin Psychol 66(2):423–428, 1998 9583345

Bloch MH, Bartley CA, Zipperer L, et al: Meta-analysis: hoarding symptoms associated with poor treatment outcome in obsessive-compulsive disorder. Mol Psychiatry 19(9):1025–1030, 2014 24912494

Calvo R, Lázaro L, Castro-Fornieles J, et al: Obsessive-compulsive personality disorder traits and personality dimensions in parents of children with obsessive-compulsive disorder. Eur Psychiatry 24(3):201–206, 2009 19118984

Cavedini P, Erzegovesi S, Ronchi P, Bellodi L: Predictive value of obsessive-compulsive personality disorder in antiobsessional pharmacological treatment. Eur Neuropsychopharmacol 7(1):45–49, 1997 9088884

Coles ME, Pinto A, Mancebo MC, et al: OCD with comorbid OCPD: a subtype of OCD? J Psychiatr Res 42(4):289–296, 2008 17382961

Diedrich A, Voderholzer U: Obsessive-compulsive personality disorder: a current review. Curr Psychiatry Rep 17(2):2, 2015 25617042

Ecker W, Kupfer J, Gönner S: Incompleteness as a link between obsessive-compulsive personality traits and specific symptom dimensions of obsessive-compulsive disorder. Clin Psychol Psychother 21(5):394–402, 2014 23650140

Egan SJ, Wade TD, Shafran R: Perfectionism as a transdiagnostic process: a clinical review. Clin Psychol Rev 31(2):203–212, 2011 20488598

Egan SJ, Piek JP, Dyck MJ, et al: A clinical investigation of motivation to change standards and cognitions about failure in perfectionism. Behav Cogn Psychother 41(5):565–578, 2013 23043771

Eisen JL, Coles ME, Shea MT, et al: Clarifying the convergence between obsessive compulsive personality disorder criteria and obsessive compulsive disorder. J Pers Disord 20(3):294–305, 2006 16776557

Fairburn CG, Cooper Z, Shafran R: Cognitive behaviour therapy for eating disorders: a "transdiagnostic" theory and treatment. Behav Res Ther 41(5):509–528, 2003 12711261

Fossati A, Beauchaine TP, Grazioli F, et al: Confirmatory factor analyses of DSM-IV Cluster C personality disorder criteria. J Pers Disord 20(2):186–203, 2006 16643123

Freud S: Character and anal eroticism(1908), in Standard Edition of the Complete Psychological Works of Sigmund Freud, Vol 9. Translated and edited by Strachey J. London, Hogarth Press, 1959, pp 167–176

Frost RO, Gross RC: The hoarding of possessions. Behav Res Ther 31(4):367–381, 1993 8512538

Frost RO, Marten P, Lahart C, et al: The dimensions of perfectionism. Cognit Ther Res 14(5):449–468, 1990

Frost RO, Steketee G, Cohn L, et al: Personality traits in subclinical and non-obsessive-compulsive volunteers and their parents. Behav Res Ther 32(1):47–56, 1994 8135722

Frost RO, Steketee G, Tolin DF: Comorbidity in hoarding disorder. Depress Anxiety 28(10):876–884, 2011 21770000

Gilliam CM, Norberg MM, Villavicencio A, et al: Group cognitive-behavioral therapy for hoarding disorder: an open trial. Behav Res Ther 49(11):802–807, 2011 21925643

Goodman WK, Price LH, Rasmussen SA, et al: The Yale-Brown Obsessive Compulsive Scale: I. Development, use, and reliability. Arch Gen Psychiatry 46(11):1006–1011, 1989 2684084

Gordon OM, Salkovskis PM, Bream V: The impact of obsessive compulsive personality disorder on cognitive behaviour therapy for obsessive compulsive disorder. Behav Cogn Psychother 44(4):444–459, 2016 27246860

Grant JE, Mooney ME, Kushner MG: Prevalence, correlates, and comorbidity of DSM-IV obsessive-compulsive personality disorder: results from the National Epidemiologic Survey on Alcohol and Related Conditions. J Psychiatr Res 46(4):469–475, 2012 22257387

Gunderson JG, Shea MT, Skodol AE, et al: The Collaborative Longitudinal Personality Disorders Study: development, aims, design, and sample characteristics. J Pers Disord 14(4):300–315, 2000 11213788

Janet P: Les Obsessions et la Psychasthenie, 2nd Edition. Paris, Bailliere, 1904

Koran L, Simpson H: Guideline Watch (March 2013): practice guideline for the treatment of patients with obsessive-compulsive disorder. 2013. Available at: https://psychiatryonline.org/pb/assets/raw/sitewide/practice_guidelines/guidelines/ocd-watch.pdf. Accessed April 9, 2019.

Kyrios M, Hordern C, Fassnacht DB: Predictors of response to cognitive behaviour therapy for obsessive-compulsive disorder. Int J Clin Health Psychol 15(3):181–190, 2015 30487835

Landau D, Iervolino AC, Pertusa A, et al: Stressful life events and material deprivation in hoarding disorder. J Anxiety Disord 25(2):192–202, 2011 20934847

Lenane MC, Swedo SE, Leonard H, et al: Psychiatric disorders in first degree relatives of children and adolescents with obsessive compulsive disorder. J Am Acad Child Adolesc Psychiatry 29(3):407–412, 1990 2347838

Mataix-Cols D, Frost RO, Pertusa A, et al: Hoarding disorder: a new diagnosis for DSM-V? Depress Anxiety 27(6):556–572, 2010 20336805

McGlashan TH, Grilo CM, Skodol AE, et al: The Collaborative Longitudinal Personality Disorders Study: baseline Axis I/II and II/II diagnostic co-occurrence. Acta Psychiatr Scand 102(4):256–264, 2000 11089725

McGlashan TH, Grilo CM, Sanislow CA, et al: Two-year prevalence and stability of individual DSM-IV criteria for schizotypal, borderline, avoidant, and obsessive-compulsive personality disorders: toward a hybrid model of axis II disorders. Am J Psychiatry 162(5):883–889, 2005 15863789

Muroff J, Steketee G, Frost RO, et al: Cognitive behavior therapy for hoarding disorder: follow-up findings and predictors of outcome. Depress Anxiety 31(12):964–971, 2014 24277161

Murray CJ, Lopez AD, World Health Organization, et al: The Global Burden of Disease: A Comprehensive Assessment of Mortality and Disability From Diseases, Injuries, and Risk Factors in 1990 and Projected to 2020: Summary. Geneva, World Health Organization, 1996

Obsessive Compulsive Cognitions Working Group: Cognitive assessment of obsessive-compulsive disorder. Behav Res Ther 35(7):667–681, 1997 9193129

Obsessive Compulsive Cognitions Working Group: Psychometric validation of the Obsessive Belief Questionnaire and interpretation of intrusions inventory—Part 2: Factor analyses and testing of a brief version. Behav Res Ther 43(11):1527–1542, 2005 16299894

O'Connor RC: The relations between perfectionism and suicidality: a systematic review. Suicide Life Threat Behav 37(6):698–714, 2007 18275376

Park JM, Storch EA, Pinto A, et al: Obsessive-compulsive personality traits in youth with obsessive-compulsive disorder. Child Psychiatry Hum Dev 47(2):281–290, 2016 26160348

Pfohl B, Blum N, Zimmerman M, et al: Structured Interview for DSM-III-R Personality (SIDP-R). Iowa City, IA, Department of Psychiatry, University of Iowa, 1989

Pinto A, Mancebo MC, Eisen JL, et al: The Brown Longitudinal Obsessive Compulsive Study: clinical features and symptoms of the sample at intake. J Clin Psychiatry 67(5):703–711, 2006 16841619

Pinto A, Liebowitz MR, Foa EB, et al: Obsessive compulsive personality disorder as a predictor of exposure and ritual prevention outcome for obsessive compulsive disorder. Behav Res Ther 49(8):453–458, 2011 21600563

Pinto A, Steinglass JE, Greene AL, et al: Capacity to delay reward differentiates obsessive-compulsive disorder and obsessive-compulsive personality disorder. Biol Psychiatry 75(8):653–659, 2014 24199665

Pinto A, Greene AL, Storch EA, et al: Prevalence of childhood obsessive-compulsive personality traits in adults with obsessive compulsive disorder versus obsessive compulsive personality disorder. J Obsessive Compuls Relat Disord 4:25–29, 2015 25574456

Pinto A, Dargani N, Wheaton MG, et al: Perfectionism in obsessive-compulsive disorder and related disorders: what should treating clinicians know? J Obsessive Compuls Relat Disord 12:102–108, 2017

Pinto A, Ansell E, Wheaton MG, et al: Obsessive compulsive personality disorder and its component personality traits, in Handbook of Personality Disorders, 2nd Edition. Edited by Livesley W, Larstone R. New York, Guilford, 2018, pp 459–480

Rhéaume J, Freeston MH, Dugas MJ, et al: Perfectionism, responsibility and obsessive-compulsive symptoms. Behav Res Ther 33(7):785–794, 1995 7677716

Rice KG, Aldea MA: State dependence and trait stability of perfectionism: a short-term longitudinal study. J Couns Psychol 53:205–212, 2006

Ruscio AM, Stein DJ, Chiu WT, et al: The epidemiology of obsessive-compulsive disorder in the National Comorbidity Survey Replication. Mol Psychiatry 15(1):53–63, 2010 18725912

Samuels J, Nestadt G, Bienvenu OJ, et al: Personality disorders and normal personality dimensions in obsessive-compulsive disorder. Br J Psychiatry 177:457–462, 2000 11060001

Shea MT, Stout RL, Yen S, et al: Associations in the course of personality disorders and Axis I disorders over time. J Abnorm Psychol 113(4):499–508, 2004 15535783

Skapinakis P, Caldwell DM, Hollingworth W, et al: Pharmacological and psychotherapeutic interventions for management of obsessive-compulsive disorder in adults: a systematic review and network meta-analysis. Lancet Psychiatry 3(8):730–739, 2016 27318812

Southgate L, Tchanturia K, Collier D, et al: The development of the Childhood Retrospective Perfectionism Questionnaire (CHIRP) in an eating disorder sample. Eur Eat Disord Rev 16(6):451–462, 2008 18444228

Starcevic V, Brakoulias V: New diagnostic perspectives on obsessive-compulsive personality disorder and its links with other conditions. Curr Opin Psychiatry 27(1):62–67, 2014 24257122

Starcevic V, Berle D, Brakoulias V, et al: Obsessive-compulsive personality disorder co-occurring with obsessive-compulsive disorder: conceptual and clinical implications. Aust NZ J Psychiatry 47(1):65–73, 2013 22689335

Steketee G, Frost RO, Kyrios M: Cognitive aspects of compulsive hoarding. Cognit Ther Res 27(4):463–479, 2003

Steketee G, Frost RO, Tolin DF, et al: Waitlist-controlled trial of cognitive behavior therapy for hoarding disorder. Depress Anxiety 27(5):476–484, 2010 20336804

Stoeber J: Multidimensional perfectionism and the DSM-5 personality traits. Pers Individ Dif 64:115–120, 2014

Summerfeldt LJ: Understanding and treating incompleteness in obsessive-compulsive disorder. J Clin Psychol 60(11):1155–1168, 2004 15389620

Swedo SE, Rapoport JL, Leonard H, et al: Obsessive-compulsive disorder in children and adolescents: clinical phenomenology of 70 consecutive cases. Arch Gen Psychiatry 46(4):335–341, 1989 2930330

Thomsen PH, Mikkelsen HU: Development of personality disorders in children and adolescents with obsessive-compulsive disorder: a 6- to 22-year follow-up study. Acta Psychiatr Scand 87(6):456–462, 1993 8356899

Wheaton MG, Pinto A: Obsessive-compulsive personality disorder, in The Wiley Handbook of Obsessive-Compulsive Disorders. Edited by McKay D, Storch EA, Abramowitz JS. Hoboken, NJ, Wiley-Blackwell, 2017, pp 726–742

Wheaton MG, Abramowitz JS, Fabricant LE, et al: Is hoarding a symptom of obsessive-compulsive disorder? Int J Cogn Ther 4(3):225–238, 2011

Widiger TA: Dimensional models of personality disorder. World Psychiatry 6(2):79–83, 2007 18235857

Widiger TA, Sanderson CJ: Toward a dimensional model of personality disorders, in Diagnosis and Treatment of Mental Disorders: The DSM-IV Personality Disorders. Edited by Livesley WJ. New York, Guilford, 1995, pp 433–458

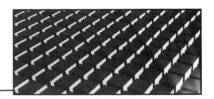

CHAPTER 4

OCPD AND ITS RELATIONSHIP TO EATING DISORDERS

Kaitlyn Wright, B.A.

Scott J. Crow, M.D.

Case Vignette

Catherine is a 26-year-old female. She works as a paralegal at a law firm and is often distracted during work because of her intense calorie counting and fear of others watching her eat. She often finds an excuse when her coworkers invite her to join them for lunch. Catherine also becomes frustrated with them when they do not organize things in the system that Catherine prefers. She is perfectionistic, and when she is not thinking about calories, she spends much of her day concerned about the way in which things are being done in the office, so much so that she often does not finish tasks that have been assigned to her. This behavior has been to the detriment of her relationships with her coworkers. Catherine's boss has tried to discuss this with her, but her rigid nature makes it difficult for her to understand why no one understands that her solution is the best.

Outside of work, Catherine lives with two of her friends. In recent months, Catherine has spent less time with them because she is focused

71

on work and staying in strict control of her weight. Catherine's roommates have tried to talk to her about making time for herself and her
friends, but she only argues that she is devoted to her work.

Within the past 6 months, Catherine's weight has dropped from
145 pounds to 111 pounds. She is 5'7" and now has a body mass index
(BMI) of 17.4. Catherine was hospitalized 2 months ago and was admitted to a treatment program, but she has yet to make any significant
gains in her recovery. She describes a fear of gaining weight and reports
that she needs to lose at least 4 more pounds in order to be viewed as
perfect by her friends and coworkers. She counts her calories very
strictly, aiming for 500 per day.

Eating disorders (anorexia nervosa, bulimia nervosa, binge-eating
disorder, avoidant/restrictive food intake disorder, and other specified
feeding or eating disorders) are serious and potentially life-threatening
mental health conditions. Eating disorders often emerge during adolescence (Allen et al. 2013). Using results from the National Comorbidity
Survey Replication, Hudson et al. (2007) found that anorexia nervosa
affects approximately 0.9% of females and 0.3% of males; bulimia nervosa affects 1.5% of females and 0.5% of males; and binge eating affects
3.5% of females and 2.0% of males. Eating disorders are characterized
by a disturbance in body image that manifests in a variety of symptoms
and risk factors, affecting both onset and treatment of eating disorders.
Individuals with eating disorders typically exhibit abnormalities in eating habits as well as a strong discomfort with their own weight and/or
shape. Individuals often experience diagnostic crossover, in which
symptoms may be represented across multiple eating disorder diagnoses (Askew and Haynos, in press). Eating disorders also have a significant impact on an individual's psychosocial functioning (e.g.,
depression, anxiety, poor social interaction). Indeed, they are associated
with an increased risk of self-harm behaviors, suicide attempts, and a
multitude of other mental health concerns (Favaro et al. 2007; Welch
and Fairburn 1996).

Although eating disorders affect a significant percentage of the population, disordered eating is even more prevalent. Disordered eating is
a separate diagnostic category (other specified feeding or eating disorder [OSFED]) that classifies individuals who have disturbances in eating behaviors and weight and shape concerns but do not meet the full
diagnostic criteria for other eating disorders. In addition, OSFED is associated with many of the same risk factors as eating disorders, such as
increased substance use and high mortality rates (Crow et al. 2009;
Pisetsky et al. 2008). OSFED represents a similar pattern of high comorbidity as seen in other eating disorders (Fairburn et al. 2007).

Emerging research over the past several decades has shown consistent evidence of the co-occurrence of eating disorders and personality

disorders (Rosenvinge et al. 2000; Sansone and Sansone 2011). There is overall consensus that personality disorders in individuals with eating disorders are of significant concern, given that personality disorders are more prevalent in people with eating disorder pathology than in the general population. However, researchers have found varying rates of comorbidity between obsessive-compulsive personality disorder (OCPD) and eating disorders. For example, von Lojewski and Abraham (2014) found rates of personality disorders among individuals with eating disorders to be approximately 21%. Other studies suggest rates ranging from 30% to 60% (Cassin and von Ranson 2005; Godt 2008). Serpell et al. (2002) suggested that prevalence rates differ because of varying methodology and diagnostic tools used to diagnose personality disorders. The wide variation among studies highlights the need for further understanding of the relationship between personality disorders and eating disorders. Importantly, Sansone and Sansone (2011) noted that these estimates consider only those individuals who meet full diagnostic criteria for both eating disorders and personality disorders. Estimates do not include individuals with disordered eating or individuals with personality disorder traits that may not be clinically diagnosable as a personality disorder. Therefore, the risk of comorbid personality disorders among individuals with eating disorders may be underrepresented in the literature.

The relationship between OCPD and eating disorder onset is relatively unclear. However, research indicates that OCPD precedes the onset of eating disorder symptoms and diagnosis (Matsunaga et al. 2000). More specifically, personality pathology often increases one's risk for eating disorders. The hallmark traits of OCPD may be factors that put an individual at risk for eating disorders. For example, a number of studies have suggested that personality traits seen in OCPD, especially perfectionism, may influence the risk for eating disorder symptoms (Anderluh et al. 2003; Halmi 2005; Jacobi et al. 2004). In addition, maintaining a sense of control is a core feature in both eating disorders and personality disorders and may play a significant role in the maintenance of eating disorder symptoms.

Given that recovery from eating disorders is difficult, it is important to note that all personality disorders have been found to worsen treatment outcomes and recovery in all diagnostic categories of eating disorders, including OSFED (Masheb and Grilo 2008; Rø et al. 2005). Indeed, many studies have indicated that OCPD continues after recovery from the eating disorder. This persistence of OCPD may also complicate recovery from the eating disorder and lead to poor outcomes of eating disorder treatment. One randomized controlled trial suggested that traits such as perfectionism in OCPD may serve as moderators in the recovery of eating disorders, worsening outcomes (Lock et al. 2005).

EATING DISORDERS AND OCPD

Anorexia Nervosa

Anorexia nervosa (AN) is characterized by a significantly low body weight due to a restriction of caloric intake relative to energy needs. More specifically, according to DSM-5 (American Psychiatric Association 2013), AN is determined by restriction of energy intake, relative to age, sex, and developmental trajectory, that causes significantly low weight and an intense fear of weight gain or becoming fat despite low weight. Additionally, AN is classified by a disturbance in the perception of one's weight or shape. The disturbance and fear of weight gain can be expressed in cognitive endorsements and/or behaviors. Such fears do not diminish once weight loss is achieved. AN can be divided into subtypes, including restricting type and binge-eating/purging type. AN restricting type occurs when an individual attains weight loss through restricting calories by dieting, fasting, and/or excessive exercise. Individuals with the restricting type do not engage in bingeing or purging behaviors. AN binge-eating/purging type occurs when an individual with AN engages in binge eating and/or purging (e.g., vomiting, misuse of laxatives) to attain weight loss.

AN has the highest mortality rate of any psychiatric disorder (Klump et al. 2009) and is persistent and difficult to treat. Researchers have found that adolescents with AN have a more successful rate of recovery than adults. For example, longitudinal data on adolescents with AN indicate a recovery rate of 69% (Herpertz-Dahlmann et al. 2001). However, adults with AN have a much lower recovery rate. Some studies suggest that as few as half of adults with AN will recover, and up to one-fifth will remain chronically ill for their lifetime (Steinhausen 2002; Steinhausen and Weber 2009). Ackard et al. (2014) found that among adults with eating disorders, those with AN ages 18–39 had the poorest treatment outcomes and highest rates of mortality compared with age groups of individuals younger than 18 and older than 40. In addition, patients with AN who require hospitalization have the worst treatment outcomes (Keel and Brown 2010).

Anorexia Nervosa and OCPD

AN is highly comorbid with a multitude of other psychiatric disorders (e.g., OCD, anxiety disorders, depression, substance use). Estimates of the comorbidity between AN and personality disorders are also high, and evidence suggests that comorbidity leads to greater severity of symptoms, lower lifetime BMI, greater number of hospitalizations, and earlier onset of AN (Gaudio and Ciommo 2011). Multiple researchers have suggested that OCPD occurs particularly among those with AN restricting subtype. Sansone and Sansone (2011) suggested that OCPD is present in about 22% of individuals with AN restricting subtype, and Thornton and Russell (1997) saw rates of AN with premorbid OCPD as high as 35%. In a review of OCPD and excessive exercise, Young et al. (2013) found a positive relationship between OCPD traits and excessive exercise among patients with AN. Researchers suggest that the personality traits that are common among individuals with AN (e.g., perfectionism, obsessionality, rigidity) are found concurrently in OCPD (Cassin and von Ranson 2005). Although it has been suggested that obsessionality and other characteristics common among patients with AN may be due to the effects of starvation, studies have found that such traits persist after weight restoration and might be in part a product of OCPD (Matsunaga et al. 2000; Nilsson et al. 1999). In fact, Anderluh et al. (2003) found that high levels of obsessive-compulsive personality traits (e.g., perfectionism and rigidity) in adolescent females led to a higher likelihood of developing an eating disorder.

Family studies have suggested that AN has strong genetic influences, and recent studies have shown that obsessive-compulsive personality traits that may result in OCPD also have a genetic basis (Lilenfeld et al. 1998). Additionally, Strober et al. (2007) examined genetic inheritance of anxiety disorders and found that relatives of individuals diagnosed with AN were three times more likely to develop OCPD, OCD, and generalized anxiety than were relatives of healthy control subjects with no history of an eating disorder.

Most researchers agree that OCPD may compromise treatment outcomes of AN. The presence of OCPD traits may increase difficulty in recovery, given perfectionistic and rigid attitudes toward weight gain and recovery (Bruce and Steiger 2005). Overall, traits that are associated with OCPD, such as perfectionism, may inhibit treatment outcomes for AN. For example, Crane et al. (2007), in a review of OCPD and AN outcome, and Steinhausen (2002) suggested that individuals with AN and co-occurring OCPD generally have worse outcomes than those with AN and no diagnosis of OCPD.

Bulimia Nervosa

Bulimia nervosa (BN) is defined in DSM-5 as recurrent episodes of binge eating followed by compensatory behaviors (e.g., self-induced vomiting, laxative misuse, diuretics, fasting, excessive exercise) (American Psychiatric Association 2013). To be classified as BN, bingeing and compensatory behaviors must occur on average at least once a week for 3 months, but individuals who present for BN treatment typically have had symptoms for a number of years before they seek treatment. Further, self-evaluation among individuals with BN is highly influenced by weight and shape. Last, a clinical diagnosis of BN requires that binge eating and compensatory behaviors do not occur exclusively in the context of AN. In practice, this differentiation is based largely on weight, and this distinction is made because recovery rates for individuals diagnosed with BN tend to be higher than for those with AN (Eddy et al. 2017).

Bulimia Nervosa and OCPD

BN is often associated with Cluster B personality disorders, particularly borderline personality disorder (Grilo 2002). However, Martinussen et al. (2017) found that Cluster B and Cluster C personality disorders occurred at similar rates in individuals with BN. In one sample, approximately 4% of individuals with BN also received a diagnosis of OCPD (Herzog et al. 1992), and another study found that approximately 5% had comorbid OCPD (Thornton and Russell 1997). Overall, there has been a lack of studies about BN and OCPD because much of the focus has surrounded BN and borderline personality disorder (Cassin and von Ranson 2005; Pearson et al. 2017).

Binge-Eating Disorder

Binge-eating disorder (BED) was added in DSM-5 and is characterized by episodes of binge eating, without the compensatory behaviors that are seen in BN (American Psychiatric Association 2013). A binge-eating episode is defined in DSM-5 as eating an objectively large amount of food within a short time period (usually less than 2 hours), as well as a loss of control over eating. The episode is characterized by eating much more rapidly than normal; eating until feeling uncomfortably full; eating large amounts of food when not feeling physically hungry; eating alone because of embarrassment about the quantity eaten; feeling disgusted with oneself, depressed, or guilty afterward; and experiencing marked distress due to the binge episode. To be classified as BED, binge-eating episodes must occur at least once a week for 3 months, must not be followed by any compensatory behaviors, and must not occur exclusively during the course of AN or BN.

The addition of BED as a diagnostic category in DSM-5 is important because of the high prevalence rate of individuals diagnosed with BED, as well as the multitude of both medical (e.g., type 2 diabetes) and psychiatric (e.g., mood and anxiety disorders) comorbidities found among individuals with BED (Grilo et al. 2009; Raevuori et al. 2015). Estimates of BED in the general population are approximately 2.0%–3.5% (Hudson et al. 2007). Typically, BED is found at somewhat higher rates among women than men (Spitzer et al. 1993). Treatment outcomes of individuals diagnosed with BED tend to be positive, and a variety of approaches are used. For example, in a review of randomized controlled trials for

BED treatment, Brownley et al. (2016) found that both psychological therapies (e.g., dialectical behavior therapy, interpersonal psychotherapy, behavioral weight loss) and pharmacological therapies (e.g., antidepressants, anticonvulsants, antiobesity agents) have some efficacy in reducing binge severity and addressing mood symptoms among patients with BED (Brownley et al. 2016).

Binge-Eating Disorder and OCPD

Given the relatively new diagnosis of BED in DSM-5, there is a dearth of literature surrounding OCPD and BED. In an examination of the relationship between binge severity and personality disorders, Picot and Lilenfeld (2003) found that personality disorders reliably predicted both increased severity and frequency of binges. Additionally, they found that OCPD and avoidant personality disorder were among the most frequent personality disorders in this sample, which is consistent with findings from Becker et al. (2010). Other researchers have also found higher rates of OCPD than any other personality disorder among individuals with BED (Becker et al. 2010; Grilo and McGlashan 2000). In addition, Wilfley et al. (2000) found that OCPD occurred at higher rates in patients with BED (14%) than in general psychiatric patients (6%). Becker et al. (2010) found higher rates of OCPD, as well as avoidant personality disorder, in an outpatient BED sample compared with community samples.

The high levels of OCPD in patients with BED may in part be due to the way in which individuals with BED often seek control of interpersonal traits (e.g., rigidity) and intrapersonal traits (e.g., perfectionism), which is similar to behavior seen among individuals with OCPD. Indeed, individuals with BED who are characterized as having high perfectionism and a preoccupation with details may be at a significantly higher risk for OCPD (Grilo 2004a). Ansell et al. (2008) examined factor model structures of OCPD as a potential risk to patients with BED and found that perfectionism and rigidity may be the best model of fit when targeting individuals who may be at the highest risk. In addition, Grilo et al. (2004b) found that rigidity accounted for 39.3% of the variance when examining aspects of control in OCPD and BED, and perfectionism accounted for 13.8%. It is clear that individuals with BED have higher levels of OCPD when identified with characteristics such as perfectionism, rigidity, and preoccupation with details, just as occurs in individuals with AN and OCPD.

Avoidant/Restrictive Food Intake Disorder

Avoidant/restrictive food intake disorder (ARFID) is an area of active and increasing research and clinical attention (American Psychiatric

Association 2013). Individuals with ARFID have severe picky eating, resulting in weight loss, distress, and nutritional and metabolic complications. There is evidence for elevated OCD symptoms in those with ARFID (Zickgraf et al. 2016), but the relationship (if any) of ARFID to OCPD is unexplored.

Other Specified Feeding or Eating Disorder

Eating disorder not otherwise specified (EDNOS) was added in DSM-IV (American Psychiatric Association 1994) and was the most frequently diagnosed eating disorder (Fairburn and Bohn 2005; Hay et al. 2008). In DSM-5, EDNOS was reclassified as other specified feeding or eating disorder (OSFED). Although the nosology and some aspects of the diagnostic criteria have changed, to avoid confusion, we will refer simply to OSFED rather than using both EDNOS and OSFED. OSFED impacts individuals by causing clinically significant distress, but it does not meet the clinical criteria for another eating disorder. Individuals qualify for OSFED if they experience impairment in social, occupational, or other areas of functioning in response to the impairment of feeding or eating. For example, DSM-5 provides five examples of OSFED: 1) *atypical anorexia nervosa*, in which criteria for AN are met except that the patient's weight remains within or above the normal range; 2) *bulimia nervosa of low frequency and/or limited duration*, in which criteria for BN are met except that the behaviors occur, on average, less than once a week and/or for less than 3 months; 3) *binge-eating disorder of low frequency and/or limited duration*, in which criteria for BED are met except that binge eating occurs, on average, less than once a week and/or for less than 3 months; 4) *purging disorder*, characterized by recurrent purging without binge eating; and 5) *night eating syndrome*, characterized by recurrent episodes of night eating. The addition of OSFED to DSM is critical, not only because of the high prevalence rates, but also because individuals with OSFED are frequently reported to have levels of psychopathology similar to those of AN and BN, as well as elevated mortality rates (Crow et al. 2009; Thomas et al. 2009).

OSFED often appears in adolescence, and this population experiences disordered eating at higher rates than occur in the general population. Approximately 2.7%–4.1% of females and 0.6%–0.9% of males receive a diagnosis of OSFED (Allen et al. 2013). Individuals may be diagnosed with OSFED before they are diagnosed with a full eating disorder or as they recover from a full eating disorder. However, individuals may also be diagnosed with OSFED without ever reaching full criteria. OSFED also has a more positive rate of recovery than do AN and BN (Ben-Tovim et al. 2001). In a study of OSFED and recovery rates, Agras et al. (2009) found that approximately 80% of individuals recovered from OSFED within 4 years of diagnosis.

Similar to BED, OSFED as a clinical category of eating disorders is important given the high prevalence of comorbid personality disorders. Although few studies to date have examined the relationship between personality disorders and disordered eating behaviors, data suggest that individuals with OSFED face a similar prevalence rate of co-occurring personality disorders as seen in other eating disorders. For instance, Raynal et al. (2016) found that individuals with disordered eating behaviors had a higher likelihood of personality disorder traits compared with healthy controls. Although studies examining OCPD and OSFED are limited, some studies have indicated that OCPD and disordered eating have similar outcomes to other eating disorders and OCPD. Perkins et al. (2013) examined three personality clusters—adaptive, rigid, and dysregulated—among a sample of females with disordered eating pathology. Similar to findings among individuals with clinical levels of AN (restricting and binge-eating/purging type) and BN, Perkins and colleagues found that that 60% of females with disordered eating had the highest levels of adaptive cluster traits (i.e., perfectionistic) and that those with BN had the highest level of dysregulated cluster traits (i.e., impulsive). Importantly, they also found that disordered eating and the co-occurrence of personality clusters significantly predicted social functioning. Therefore, it is clear that individuals with OSFED and co-occurring personality disorders—specifically, traits that align with OCPD—have a risk profile similar to that of individuals who experience full-blown eating disorders.

FUTURE DIRECTIONS FOR RESEARCH

Research to date has provided some insight into the relationship between OCPD and eating disorders, specifically in regard to prevalence rates and poor outcome results for individuals with OCPD and eating disorders. However, significant gaps in the current research on OCPD and eating disorders exist in the literature. Future research should examine the relationships between the onset of OCPD and eating disorders to determine the specific causal mechanisms underlying the high comorbidity rates observed. In addition, it would be important to understand treatment for the co-occurrence of the disorders because both present challenges to recovery and the possibility of future relapse.

Returning to our case study, it is clear that Catherine suffers from the co-occurrence of OCPD and AN. She is preoccupied with perfectionism such that the major point of the activity is lost in her work, she is unable to complete her work, and she is devoted to work to the point of losing relationships. Catherine also meets criteria for AN. She has an intense fear of weight gain, and weight has an undue influence on her self-evaluation. In addition, Catherine refuses to gain weight and weighs less than 85% of the weight expected for her age and height.

TAKE-HOME POINTS

- Eating disorders are serious mental health conditions that can be life-threatening.
- The co-occurrence of eating disorders and OCPD is high.
- AN restricting type may be most severely impacted by OCPD.
- OCPD worsens treatment outcomes and recovery in all diagnostic categories of eating disorders.

REFERENCES

Ackard DM, Richter S, Egan A, et al: Poor outcome and death among youth, young adults, and midlife adults with eating disorders: an investigation of risk factors by age at assessment. Int J Eat Disord 47(7):825–835, 2014 25111891

Agras WS, Crow S, Mitchell JE, et al: A 4-year prospective study of eating disorder NOS compared with full eating disorder syndromes. Int J Eat Disord 42(6):565–570, 2009 19544557

Allen KL, Byrne SM, Oddy WH, et al: DSM-IV-TR and DSM-5 eating disorders in adolescents: prevalence, stability, and psychosocial correlates in a population-based sample of male and female adolescents. J Abnorm Psychol 122(3):720–732, 2013 24016012

American Psychiatric Association: Diagnostic and Statistical Manual of Mental Disorders, 4th Edition. Washington, DC, American Psychiatric Association, 1994

American Psychiatric Association: Diagnostic and Statistical Manual of Mental Disorders, 5th Edition. Arlington, VA, American Psychiatric Publishing, 2013

Anderluh MB, Tchanturia K, Rabe-Hesketh S, et al: Childhood obsessive-compulsive personality traits in adult women with eating disorders: defining a broader eating disorder phenotype. Am J Psychiatry 160(2):242–247, 2003 12562569

Ansell EB, Pinto A, Edelen MO, Grillo CM: Structure of Diagnostic and Statistical Manual of Mental Disorders, Fourth Edition criteria for obsessive-compulsive personality disorder in patients with binge eating disorder. Can J Psychiatry 53(12):863–867, 2008 19087485

Askew A, Haynos AF: Eating disorders, in The Encyclopedia of Child and Adolescent Development. Edited by Hupp S, Jewell J. Hoboken, NJ, Wiley-Blackwell (in press)

Becker DF, Masheb RM, White MA, et al: Psychiatric, behavioral, and attitudinal correlates of avoidant and obsessive-compulsive personality pathology in patients with binge-eating disorder. Compr Psychiatry 51(5):531–537, 2010 20728012

Ben-Tovim DI, Walker K, Gilchrist P, et al: Outcome in patients with eating disorders: a 5-year study. Lancet 357(9264):1254–1257, 2001 11418150

Brownley KA, Berkman ND, Peat CM, et al: Binge-eating disorder in adults: a systematic review and meta-analysis. Ann Intern Med 165(6):409–420, 2016 27367316

Bruce KR, Steiger H: Treatment implications of Axis-II comorbidity in eating disorders. Eat Disord 13(1):93–108, 2005 16864334

Cassin SE, von Ranson KM: Personality and eating disorders: a decade in review. Clin Psychol Rev 25(7):895–916, 2005 16099563

Crane AM, Roberts ME, Treasure J: Are obsessive-compulsive personality traits associated with a poor outcome in anorexia nervosa? A systematic review of randomized controlled trials and naturalistic outcome studies. Int J Eat Disord 40(7):581–588, 2007 17607713

Crow SJ, Peterson CB, Swanson SA, et al: Increased mortality in bulimia nervosa and other eating disorders. Am J Psychiatry 166(12):1342–1346, 2009 19833789

Eddy KT, Tabri N, Thomas JJ, et al: Recovery from anorexia nervosa and bulimia nervosa at 22-year follow-up. J Clin Psychiatry 78(2):184–189, 2017 28002660

Fairburn CG, Bohn K: Eating disorder NOS (EDNOS): an example of the troublesome "not otherwise specified" (NOS) category in DSM-IV. Behav Res Ther 43(6):691–701, 2005 15890163

Fairburn CG, Cooper Z, Bohn K, et al: The severity and status of eating disorder NOS: implications for DSM-V. Behav Res Ther 45(8):1705–1715, 2007 17374360

Favaro A, Ferrara S, Santonastaso P: Self-injurious behavior in a community sample of young women: relationship with childhood abuse and other types of self-damaging behaviors. J Clin Psychiatry 68(1):122–131, 2007 17284140

Gaudio S, Di Ciommo V: Prevalence of personality disorders and their clinical correlates in outpatient adolescents with anorexia nervosa. Psychosom Med 73(9):769–774, 2011 22042882

Godt K: Personality disorders in 545 patients with eating disorders. Eur Eat Disord Rev 16(2):94–99, 2008 18059070

Grilo CM: Recent research of relationships among eating disorders and personality disorders. Curr Psychiatry Rep 4(1):18–24, 2002 11814391

Grilo CM: Diagnostic efficiency of DSM-IV criteria for obsessive compulsive personality disorder in patients with binge eating disorder. Behav Res Ther 42(1):57–65, 2004a 14744523

Grilo CM: Factor structure of DSM-IV criteria for obsessive compulsive personality disorder in patients with binge eating disorder. Acta Psychiatr Scand 109(1):64–69, 2004b 14674960

Grilo CM, McGlashan TH: Convergent and discriminant validity of DSM-IV axis II personality disorder criteria in adult outpatients with binge eating disorder. Compr Psychiatry 41(3):163–166, 2000 10834623

Grilo CM, White MA, Masheb RM: DSM-IV psychiatric disorder comorbidity and its correlates in binge eating disorder. Int J Eat Disord 42(3):228–234, 2009 18951458

Halmi KA: Obsessive-compulsive personality disorder and eating disorders. Eat Disord 13(1):85–92, 2005 16864333

Hay PJ, Mond J, Buttner P, et al: Eating disorder behaviors are increasing: findings from two sequential community surveys in South Australia. PLoS One 3(2):e1541, 2008 18253489

Herpertz-Dahlmann B, Müller B, Herpertz S, et al: Prospective 10-year follow-up in adolescent anorexia nervosa: course, outcome, psychiatric comorbidity, and psychosocial adaptation. J Child Psychol Psychiatry 42(5):603–612, 2001 11464965

Herzog DB, Keller MB, Lavori PW, et al: The prevalence of personality disorders in 210 women with eating disorders. J Clin Psychiatry 53(5):147–152, 1992 1592839

Hudson JI, Hiripi E, Pope HG Jr, et al: The prevalence and correlates of eating disorders in the National Comorbidity Survey Replication. Biol Psychiatry 61(3):348–358, 2007 16815322

Jacobi C, Hayward C, de Zwaan M, et al: Coming to terms with risk factors for eating disorders: application of risk terminology and suggestions for a general taxonomy. Psychol Bull 130(1):19–65, 2004 14717649

Keel PK, Brown TA: Update on course and outcome in eating disorders. Int J Eat Disord 43(3):195–204, 2010 20186717

Klump KL, Bulik CM, Kaye WH, et al: Academy for eating disorders position paper: eating disorders are serious mental illnesses. Int J Eat Disord 42(2):97–103, 2009 18951455

Lilenfeld LR, Kaye WH, Greeno CG, et al: A controlled family study of anorexia nervosa and bulimia nervosa: psychiatric disorders in first-degree relatives and effects of proband comorbidity. Arch Gen Psychiatry 55(7):603–610, 1998 9672050

Lock J, Agras WS, Bryson S, et al: A comparison of short- and long-term family therapy for adolescent anorexia nervosa. J Am Acad Child Adolesc Psychiatry 44(7):632–639, 2005 15968231

Martinussen M, Friborg O, Schmierer P, et al: The comorbidity of personality disorders in eating disorders: a meta-analysis. Eat Weight Disord 22(2):201–209, 2017 27995489

Masheb RM, Grilo CM: Examination of predictors and moderators for self-help treatments of binge-eating disorder. J Consult Clin Psychol 76(5):900–904, 2008 18837607

Matsunaga H, Kaye WH, McConaha C, et al: Personality disorders among subjects recovered from eating disorders. Int J Eat Disord 27(3):353–357, 2000 10694723

Nilsson EW, Gillberg C, Gillberg IC, Rastam M: Ten-year follow-up of adolescent-onset anorexia nervosa: personality disorders. J Am Acad Child Adolesc Psychiatry 38(11):1389–1395, 1999 10560225

Pearson CM, Lavender JM, Cao L, et al: Associations of borderline personality disorder traits with stressful events and emotional reactivity in women with bulimia nervosa. J Abnorm Psychol 126(5):531–539, 2017 28691843

Perkins PS, Slane JD, Klump KL: Personality clusters and family relationships in women with disordered eating symptoms. Eat Behav 14(3):299–308, 2013 23910771

Picot AK, Lilenfeld LR: The relationship among binge severity, personality psychopathology, and body mass index. Int J Eat Disord 34(1):98–107, 2003 12772174

Pisetsky EM, Chao YM, Dierker LC, et al: Disordered eating and substance use in high-school students: results from the Youth Risk Behavior Surveillance System. Int J Eat Disord 41(5):464–470, 2008 18348283

Raevuori A, Suokas J, Haukka J, et al: Highly increased risk of type 2 diabetes in patients with binge eating disorder and bulimia nervosa. Int J Eat Disord 48(6):555–562, 2015 25060427

Raynal P, Melioli T, Chabrol H: Personality profiles in young adults with disordered eating behavior. Eat Behav 22:119–123, 2016 27289047

Rø O, Martinsen EW, Hoffart A, et al: Two-year prospective study of personality disorders in adults with longstanding eating disorders. Int J Eat Disord 37(2):112–118, 2005 15732071

Rosenvinge JH, Martinussen M, Østensen E: The comorbidity of eating disorders and personality disorders: a meta-analytic review of studies published between 1983 and 1998. Eat Weight Disord 5(2):52–61, 2000 10941603

Sansone RA, Sansone LA: Personality pathology and its influence on eating disorders. Innov Clin Neurosci 8(3):14–18, 2011 21487541

Serpell L, Livingston A, Neiderman M, Lask B: Anorexia nervosa: obsessive-compulsive disorder, obsessive-compulsive personality disorder, or neither? Clin Psychol Rev 22(5):647–669, 2002 12113200

Spitzer RL, Yanovski S, Wadden T, et al: Binge eating disorder: its further validation in a multisite study. Int J Eat Disord 13(2):137–153, 1993 8477283

Steinhausen HC: The outcome of anorexia nervosa in the 20th century. Am J Psychiatry 159(8):1284–1293, 2002 12153817

Steinhausen HC, Weber S: The outcome of bulimia nervosa: findings from one-quarter century of research. Am J Psychiatry 166(12):1331–1341, 2009 19884225

Strober M, Freemen R, Lampert C, Diamond J: The association of anxiety disorders and obsessive compulsive personality disorder with anorexia nervosa: evidence from a family study with discussion of nosological and neurodevelopmental implications. Int J Eat Disord 40(suppl):S46–S51, 2007 17610248

Thomas JJ, Vartanian LR, Brownell KD: The relationship between eating disorder not otherwise specified (EDNOS) and officially recognized eating disorders: meta-analysis and implications for DSM. Psychol Bull 135(3):407–433, 2009 19379023

Thornton C, Russell J: Obsessive compulsive comorbidity in the dieting disorders. Int J Eat Disord 21(1):83–87, 1997 8986521

von Lojewski A, Abraham S: Personality factors and eating disorders: self-uncertainty. Eat Behav 15(1):106–109, 2014 24411761

Welch SL, Fairburn CG: Impulsivity or comorbidity in bulimia nervosa: a controlled study of deliberate self-harm and alcohol and drug misuse in a community sample. Br J Psychiatry 169(4):451–458, 1996 8894196

Wilfley DE, Friedman MA, Dounchis JZ, et al: Comorbid psychopathology in binge eating disorder: relation to eating disorder severity at baseline and following treatment. J Consult Clin Psychol 68(4):641–649, 2000 10965639

Young S, Rhodes P, Touyz S, Hay P: The relationship between obsessive-compulsive personality disorder traits, obsessive-compulsive disorder and excessive exercise in patients with anorexia nervosa: a systematic review. J Eat Disord 1:16, 2013 24999397

Zickgraf HF, Franklin ME, Rozin P: Adult picky eaters with symptoms of avoidant/restrictive food intake disorder: comparable distress and comorbidity but different eating behaviors compared to those with disordered eating symptoms. J Eat Disord 4:26, 2016 27800160

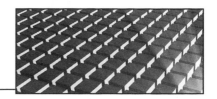

CHAPTER 5

OCPD AND ITS RELATIONSHIP TO IMPULSIVITY AND IMPULSE-CONTROL DISORDERS

Jon E. Grant, M.D., M.P.H., J.D.

Samuel R. Chamberlain, M.B./B.Chir., Ph.D., M.R.C.Psych.

Case Vignette

Robert is a 42-year-old man who comes to the clinic seeking help for his sexual behavior. He feels the behavior is compulsive in that he spends hours each day looking for sexual contacts online and the behavior interferes with his work (not being attentive at work, not meeting deadlines). He finds the sexual behavior exciting and looks forward to getting online, but after a sexual encounter he usually feels unfulfilled, ashamed of himself, and out of control.

Psychiatric examination finds that Robert has no significant mood symptoms and no other addictive behaviors, but it clearly reveals a personality profile of perfectionism (his home is spotless and no one is allowed in it), rigidity (friends tell him that he cannot compromise in anything), hypermorality (he recognizes the irony of this quality, but he judges others harshly and feels there are definite right and wrong behaviors and values), and miserliness (he will go to great lengths to save a few pennies even though his salary is well above average and he has savings and investments). His problems have ruined interpersonal relationships and left him bitter and lonely.

Obsessive-compulsive personality disorder (OCPD) is characterized by a strong desire for perfectionism, control, and orderliness, and individuals with OCPD tend to present with inflexibility, rigidity, and stubbornness (American Psychiatric Association 2013). This behavioral pattern is often associated with a lower quality of life and problems in overall psychosocial functioning (Diedrich and Voderholzer 2015; Mancebo et al. 2005; Pinto et al. 2014). In addition, OCPD is correlated with increased health costs (Bender et al. 2001, 2006; Diedrich and Voderholzer 2015; Fineberg et al. 2014; Sansone et al. 2003, 2004).

CLASSIFICATION OF OCPD

Two concepts that are of particular relevance when considering OCPD, in terms of its diagnostic classification and relationship with other disorders, are compulsivity and impulsivity. *Compulsivity* refers to repetitive, habitual actions (or mental acts) that continue despite the original goal of the task being lost and/or despite untoward longer-term consequences (Gillan et al. 2016; van den Heuvel et al. 2016). *Impulsivity* refers to behaviors that are risky, hasty, unduly thought out, or premature that result in untoward longer-term outcomes (Chamberlain and Sahakian 2007). Both compulsivity and impulsivity can be considered at the level of overt symptoms and behavior or at the level of neurocognitive functioning. Although OCPD is currently listed as a personality disorder, many researchers have thought that it has parallels with the archetypal compulsive disorder, namely, obsessive-compulsive disorder (OCD), which is now included in DSM-5 as one of the obsessive-compulsive and related disorders (American Psychiatric Association 2013).

RELATIONSHIP OF OCPD TO OCD

The relationship between OCPD and OCD has been the subject of considerable debate (Fineberg et al. 2007). OCD is characterized by obsessions (recurrent, intrusive thoughts) and/or compulsions (repetitive, unwanted behaviors), often revolving around key themes such as harm and uncertainty (Fineberg et al. 2007). It was traditionally thought that OCPD might lead to, or be causally implicated in, OCD (Gordon et al. 2013). From the perspective of top-level symptoms, individuals with OCPD and those with OCD may show rigidity in terms of tendencies to get stuck within a particular behavioral routine (Fineberg et al. 2007). Studies have reported co-occurrence of OCPD and OCD, based on more recent DSM conceptualizations, to be between 23% and 47%. In a sample of 238 treatment-seeking individuals with OCD, for example, 27% met criteria for comorbid OCPD (Coles et al. 2008). Another study, including 148 adults with OCD, found OCPD in 47.3% of the sample, and OCPD was associated with more prominent OCD symptoms (except for contamination and checking) and more distress (Starcevic et al. 2013). In a study of 403 people with OCD, comorbid OCPD occurred in 34% of the cases (Lochner et al. 2011). In a large cohort of participants in the Collaborative Longitudinal Personality Disorders Study, there was a significant association between OCPD and OCD (odds ratios of around 3), and relationships between OCPD and anxiety or mood disorders were not as strong (Eisen et al. 2006). One review that was based on OCD clinical samples found that the majority of individuals with OCD (75%) do not have OCPD. Similarly, results from personality disorder samples suggest that the majority of individuals with OCPD (80%) do not have OCD (Mancebo et al. 2005). Although not all studies agree on the high comorbidity rates, OCPD also appears to be more common in relatives of people with OCD than in relatives of control probands, hinting at a familial and possibly genetic overlap with regard to etiology (Samuels et al. 2000).

COMPULSIVITY IN INDIVIDUALS WITH OCPD

With a complicated relationship to OCD, OCPD may be better understood by considering its underlying neurocognitive similarities to OCD. To do that, it may be best to examine compulsivity in individuals with OCPD. As stated in the previous section, *compulsivity* has been defined as a tendency toward repetitive, habitual actions, which continue despite adverse consequences (Dalley et al. 2011). Additionally, compulsivity relates to the sense of being compelled to undertake an act or getting "stuck" until a situation or act is "just right" (Sica et al. 2015).

Several characteristics—extreme perfectionism affecting task completion; excessive devotion to work; and being overly inflexible, stubborn, rigid, judgmental, and conscientious—can each be linked to a central deficiency in flexibly shifting thoughts and behavior from one topic or activity to another. Individuals with OCD often employ rigid moral reasoning in response to impersonal moral dilemmas, showing a thinking style characterized by reduced cognitive flexibility (Whitton et al. 2014). In a recent study of 21 adults with OCPD compared with control subjects, the analysis of set-shifting ability on the intra-extra dimensional task (a computerized task) showed that participants with OCPD were significantly and substantially impaired on measures related specifically to the extradimensional shift (Fineberg et al. 2015). In previous research, patients with OCD, as well as patients with other typically compulsive disorders such as body dysmorphic disorder and anorexia nervosa, have also demonstrated deficits in this cognitive domain—notably, the extradimensional shift in a group with OCD comorbid with OCPD and in patients with OCD alone (Fineberg et al. 2014; Jefferies et al. 2010; Roberts et al. 2010).

Although the data on set-shifting deficits in OCPD support the concept of an underlying compulsivity, our group recently examined 23 individuals with OCPD compared with control subjects and did not find any deficits on the intra-extra dimensional task in the OCPD group (S.R. Chamberlain and J.E. Grant, unpublished data, 2019). Taken together, these studies seem to suggest that some people with OCPD may have similarities to people with OCD even at the level of neurocognitive deficits such as those found on the intra-extra dimensional task. Having said that, there may be another subgroup, however, that does not have these same compulsive features that are seen in OCD. Collectively, the findings highlight that although particular cognitive problems may be associated with particular disorders, such deficits are not universal; therefore, in the future, deficits may be useful for subtyping purposes.

RELATIONSHIP OF OCPD TO IMPULSE-CONTROL DISORDERS

If the traditional suggestion that impulsivity and compulsivity represent polar opposites of a continuum (reflecting risk seeking and risk avoidance, respectively) is correct (Stein and Hollander 1995), one might expect people with OCPD to show low rates of impulsivity because their day-to-day symptoms suggest a rigid response style and a wish for things to be perfect and controlled rather than risky and hasty. The issue of impulsivity in OCPD has had limited scrutiny. One means of understanding whether and to what extent impulsivity plays a role in OCPD would be to examine rates of co-occurring impulsive disorders within samples of people with OCPD (as well as rates of OCPD in people with impulsive disorders).

When we analyzed the literature focusing on impulse-control disorders, we identified mixed results. Keeping in mind that the number of studies of OCPD in impulse-control disorders is rather limited, the results are nevertheless provocative (Table 5–1). Given that the rate of OCPD in the general U.S. population is typically around 7.8% (Grant et al. 2012), we see that the rates of OCPD appear much higher than the population mean among people with trichotillomania (hair-pulling disorder) and excoriation (skin-picking disorder), as well as those with compulsive sexual behavior, compulsive buying, binge-eating disorder, and gambling disorder. What makes some of these findings perhaps a bit confusing is that it has never really been clear as to whether trichotillomania and skin picking are more compulsive or impulsive (in fact, trichotillomania was switched from impulse disorders in DSM-IV to the OCD-related [i.e., compulsive] disorders in DSM-5). In addition, how impulsive are these other disorders? Gambling disorder has clearly been associated with multiple forms of impulsivity (see Hodgins et al. 2011), but less is known about sexual behavior, binge eating, and buying. (Although compulsive buying has shown some signs of cognitive impulsivity [see Derbyshire et al. 2014], compulsive sexual behavior has not exhibited these signs [Derbyshire and Grant 2015].) And if the behavioral addictions are generally associated with underlying impulsivity, and if OCPD has some relationship to these disorders, why are the rates of OCPD in Internet addiction no higher than the rates of OCPD in the general population? One caveat in relation to these findings is the relatively small number of studies. The impulse-control disorders are generally underresearched and are seldom included in screening protocols for larger population-based epidemiological studies.

RELATIONSHIP OF OCPD TO DISORDERS WITH PROMINENT IMPULSIVITY

Given the numerous issues concerning the impulse-control disorders mentioned in the previous section, perhaps examining rates of OCPD in disorders with prominent impulsivity would shed more light on the relationship of OCPD to other mental health problems. In one study including a mix of individuals who were self-referred ($n=29$) or had been clinically referred ($n=89$) because of aggression problems, OCPD was evident in 24% of the sample, but antisocial personality was evident in 52%, a considerably higher percentage (Villemarette-Pittman et al. 2004). In the case of substance use disorders, an epidemiological study of 43,093 individuals found that 28.6% of respondents with a current alcohol use disorder and 47.7% of those with a current drug use disorder had at least

TABLE 5–1. Rates of OCPD in individuals with impulse-control
            disorders

Impulse-control disorder	Rate of OCPD	Reference
Kleptomania	3.6%	Grant 2004
Trichotillomania (hair-pulling disorder)	8.3%	Christenson et al. 1992
	27%	Schlosser et al. 1994a
Excoriation (skin-picking disorder)	19%	Lochner et al. 2002
	48.4%	Neziroglu et al. 2008
Compulsive sexual behavior	15%	Raymond et al. 2003
	15%	Black et al. 1997
Compulsive buying	22%	Schlosser et al. 1994b
Binge-eating disorder	19%	Becker and Grilo 2015
Internet addiction	6.6%	Zadra et al. 2016
Gambling disorder	30%	Petry et al. 2005
Pyromania	Unknown	

Note.   Rate of obsessive-compulsive personality disorder (OCPD) in the U.S. general
population is 7.8% (Grant et al. 2012).

one personality disorder. Furthermore, OCPD was found at rates of
12.1% and 16.9% in individuals with alcohol and drug use disorders, respectively (B. F. Grant et al. 2004). In one study of 145 individuals with
substance use disorders admitted to a residential dual-diagnosis chem-
ical dependency treatment program, 82 (56.6%) met criteria for OCPD
on the basis of a structured clinical interview (Grant et al. 2011). In individuals with attention-deficit/hyperactivity disorder (ADHD), OCPD is
also a common co-occurring disorder. In one study of 78 adults with
ADHD, 78% also were diagnosed with OCPD on the basis of the Structured Clinical Interview for DSM-IV (Irastorza Eguskiza et al. 2018).

IMPULSIVITY IN INDIVIDUALS WITH OCPD

In addition to examining co-occurring impulsive problems in OCPD,
other research has investigated impulsive features (not disorders) in individuals with OCPD. Data suggest normal or lower rates of impulsivity in OCPD, at least in terms of trait questionnaires and cognitive
measures. According to behavioral and neurocognitive data, impulsivity is a multidimensional (i.e., dissociable) construct (Dalley et al. 2008).
Two major domains of impulsivity are impulsive action, evidenced by

an inability to inhibit motor responses, and impulsive choice, referring to a tendency to make risky decisions (Dalley et al. 2011; Grant and Chamberlain 2014; MacKillop et al. 2016). More specifically, impulsive action reflects an inability to inhibit a prepotent (habitual or dominant) behavioral response, whereas impulsive choice reflects a preference for immediate rewards to the detriment of long-term goals. These dissociable domains have been investigated using an array of paper-and-pencil as well as laboratory-based measures.

Two common laboratory measures of motor impulsivity (an example of deficient response inhibition, which characterizes impulsive action) are go/no-go and stop-signal tasks (Band and van Boxtel 1999). On go/no-go tasks, participants are required to suppress motor activity triggered in response to a target stimulus (i.e., after presentation of the target stimulus). Participants are asked to make a rapid motor response whenever a "go" stimulus appears onscreen (e.g., horizontal lines) but to withhold their responses when a different stimulus appears (e.g., vertical lines). The go stimulus is shown more frequently than the no-go stimulus, and as a result, participants develop a prepotent tendency to respond that requires effort to suppress. Motor impulsivity is assessed by the number of times participants incorrectly respond to a no-go trial. By contrast, stop-signal tasks measure a participant's ability to inhibit (or cancel) a motor response that has already been initiated (Aron and Poldrack 2005; Logan et al. 1984). Participants who take longer to inhibit the response (a parameter referred to as the stop-signal reaction time, typically calculated using a tracking algorithm) are said to be more impulsive.

Impulsive choice (i.e., deficient deferment of gratification) refers either to the discounting of a larger reward with increasing delay (time) or to irrational risk taking. The ability to delay gratification is typically measured using temporal discounting tasks, in which participants are required to choose between an immediate but smaller reward and a larger reward in the future (Berns et al. 2007; Laibson 1997). The more quickly the subjective value of a reward decreases over time—that is, the steeper the discounting parameter—the more impulsive the participant is said to be (Peters and Büchel 2011). Similarly, decision making can be measured using the Iowa Gambling Task (Bechara et al. 1994, 1998) or the Cambridge Gambling Task (Rogers et al. 1999).

Finally, impulsivity can also be conceptualized as an aspect of personality. An extensive literature discusses the use of self-report questionnaires, including the Barratt Impulsiveness Scale (BIS-11; Patton et al. 1995; Stanford et al. 2009), to measure trait impulsivity. BIS-11 factor scores include attentional, motor, and non-planning impulsiveness. The BIS-11 is well suited for use in the population at large and is also sensitive to the more extreme levels of impulsivity that characterize ADHD (Malloy-Diniz et al. 2007).

In the case of OCPD, the data regarding impulsivity are somewhat limited. When laboratory measures of impulsivity were used, patients with OCD with and without OCPD exhibited similar levels of impulsivity on a neurocognitive task (stop-signal task), but comorbid cases had significantly worse inflexibility on a set-shifting task, indicative of being more compulsive (Daruna and Barnes 1993). In a recent study we conducted with 25 adults with OCPD compared with control subjects (J.E. Grant and S.R. Chamberlain, unpublished data, 2019), we found that after matching for age, lifetime history of mood disorders, and current anxiety disorders, those with OCPD did not differ in cognitive measures of impulsivity using the Stop Signal Response Task (stop-signal reaction times), the Cambridge Gambling Task (quality of decision making, proportion points gambled), or the Rapid Visual Information Processing test (commission errors). A study including 25 participants with OCPD, 25 patients with OCD, and 25 healthy control subjects found that OCPD was associated with increased capacity to delay reward (i.e., less reward discounting impulsivity) (Pinto et al. 2014). In that study, reward discounting was assessed using a questionnaire; patients with OCPD with and without OCD did not differ significantly on this measure, suggesting that this measure of diminished impulsivity was associated with OCPD. Finally, in a study of 110 patients with OCD, patients with comorbid OCPD (20.9% of the sample) had lower non-planning impulsivity, as indexed by the Barratt Impulsiveness Questionnaire, than did those without comorbid OCPD (Melca et al. 2015). Taken together, these cognitive or personality studies of impulsivity may actually suggest that individuals with OCPD have normal or lower levels of impulsivity compared with control subjects, depending on the measure used.

In these examples of impulsivity and disorders with fairly prominent impulsivity, what might explain the fact that such large percentages of these individuals also meet criteria for OCPD? In fact, one might expect people with OCPD to show low rates of impulsivity: their day-to-day symptoms suggest a rigid response style and wishing for things to be perfect and controlled rather than risky and hasty. One possible explanation for this co-occurrence of disorders (both seemingly on opposite sides of the impulsive-compulsive spectrum) might be that a rigid cognitive style, seen in some people with OCPD, could theoretically predispose them toward habitual patterns of behavior, such as those seen in impulse-control disorders, which may in turn lead to problematic patterns of behaviors. Another, non-mutually exclusive, explanation could be that OCPD develops as a compensatory mechanism. It has been suggested that some individuals with disinhibition may adopt a structured personality style (OCPD, or features thereof) in order to sustain functioning in work or social spheres. Finally, it could simply be that the diagnosis of OCPD is heterogeneous and that some people with OCPD are quite compulsive in nature and have co-occurring OCD, whereas others may have impulsive features and co-occurring impulse disorders.

CASE VIGNETTE DISCUSSION

Robert, described in the case vignette at the beginning of this chapter, is more likely to seek treatment for his compulsive sexual behavior than for his OCPD. In the case of compulsive sexual behavior, a potentially useful treatment approach would be cognitive-behavioral therapy, with perhaps an emphasis on body image, and use of motivational interviewing or imaginal exposures. This psychotherapeutic approach could also be augmented with medication such as naltrexone (Derbyshire and Grant 2015). What should a clinician do if Robert wants help for the OCPD as well? If the clinician sees it as an impulsive problem, then perhaps the same approach as used for the sexual behavior could be used for the OCPD. If instead it is viewed as a compulsive problem, then a more conventional approach as is often used for OCD, such as exposure response prevention and selective serotonin reuptake inhibitors, might be used. The problem is that the possible heterogeneity of OCPD has received little research attention, and therefore treatment algorithms have not been established. (For a fuller discussion of treatment for OCPD, please Chapter 9, "Psychotherapy for OCPD," and Chapter 10, "Pharmacological Treatment of OCPD.")

TAKE-HOME POINTS

- OCPD is often associated with co-occurring compulsive as well as impulsive disorders.
- Some people with OCPD may have cognitive deficits associated with impulsivity, whereas others have deficits of compulsivity.
- Treatment approaches to OCPD have not yet been refined enough to take account of these impulsive and compulsive differences, but these concepts may suggest a fruitful approach for future interventions.

REFERENCES

American Psychiatric Association: Diagnostic and Statistical Manual of Mental Disorders, 5th Edition. Arlington, VA, American Psychiatric Association, 2013

Aron AR, Poldrack RA: The cognitive neuroscience of response inhibition: relevance for genetic research in attention-deficit/hyperactivity disorder. Biol Psychiatry 57(11):1285–1292, 2005 15950000

Band GP, van Boxtel GJ: Inhibitory motor control in stop paradigms: review and reinterpretation of neural mechanisms. Acta Psychol (Amst) 101(2–3):179–211, 1999 10344185

Bechara A, Damasio AR, Damasio H, et al: Insensitivity to future consequences following damage to human prefrontal cortex. Cognition 50(1–3):7–15, 1994 8039375

Bechara A, Damasio H, Tranel D, et al: Dissociation of working memory from decision making within the human prefrontal cortex. J Neurosci 18(1):428–437, 1998 9412519

Becker DF, Grilo CM: Comorbidity of mood and substance use disorders in patients with binge-eating disorder: associations with personality disorder and eating disorder pathology. J Psychosom Res 79(2):159–164, 2015 25700727

Bender DS, Dolan RT, Skodol AE, et al: Treatment utilization by patients with personality disorders. Am J Psychiatry 158(2):295–302, 2001 11156814

Bender DS, Skodol AE, Pagano ME, et al: Prospective assessment of treatment use by patients with personality disorders. Psychiatr Serv 57(2):254–257, 2006 16452705

Berns GS, Laibson D, Loewenstein G: Intertemporal choice—toward an integrative framework. Trends Cogn Sci 11(11):482–488, 2007 17980645

Black DW, Kehrberg LL, Flumerfelt DL, et al: Characteristics of 36 subjects reporting compulsive sexual behavior. Am J Psychiatry 154(2):243–249, 1997 9016275

Chamberlain SR, Sahakian BJ: The neuropsychiatry of impulsivity. Curr Opin Psychiatry 20(3):255–261, 2007 17415079

Christenson GA, Chernoff-Clementz E, Clementz BA: Personality and clinical characteristics in patients with trichotillomania. J Clin Psychiatry 53(11):407–413, 1992 1459972

Coles ME, Pinto A, Mancebo MC, et al: OCD with comorbid OCPD: a subtype of OCD? J Psychiatr Res 42(4):289–296, 2008 17382961

Dalley JW, Mar AC, Economidou D, et al: Neurobehavioral mechanisms of impulsivity: fronto-striatal systems and functional neurochemistry. Pharmacol Biochem Behav 90(2):250–260, 2008 18272211

Dalley JW, Everitt BJ, Robbins TW: Impulsivity, compulsivity, and top-down cognitive control. Neuron 69(4):680–694, 2011 21338879

Daruna JH, Barnes PA: A neurodevelopmental view of impulsivity, in The Impulsive Client: Theory, Research, and Treatment. Washington, DC, American Psychological Associatio,. 1993, pp 23–37

Derbyshire KL, Grant JE: Neurocognitive findings in compulsive sexual behavior: a preliminary study. J Behav Addict 4(2):35–36, 2015 26014672

Derbyshire KL, Chamberlain SR, Odlaug BL, et al: Neurocognitive functioning in compulsive buying disorder. Ann Clin Psychiatry 26(1):57–63, 2014 24501731

Diedrich A, Voderholzer U: Obsessive-compulsive personality disorder: a current review. Curr Psychiatry Rep 17(2):2, 2015 25617042

Eisen JL, Coles ME, Shea MT, et al: Clarifying the convergence between obsessive compulsive personality disorder criteria and obsessive compulsive disorder. J Pers Disord 20(3):294–305, 2006 16776557

Fineberg NA, Sharma P, Sivakumaran T, et al: Does obsessive-compulsive personality disorder belong within the obsessive-compulsive spectrum? CNS Spectr 12(6):467–482, 2007 17545957

Fineberg NA, Chamberlain SR, Goudriaan AE, et al: New developments in human neurocognition: clinical, genetic, and brain imaging correlates of impulsivity and compulsivity. CNS Spectr 19(1):69–89, 2014 24512640

Fineberg NA, Day GA, de Koenigswarter N, et al: The neuropsychology of obsessive-compulsive personality disorder: a new analysis. CNS Spectr 20(5):490–499, 2015 25776273

Gillan CM, Robbins TW, Sahakian BJ, et al: The role of habit in compulsivity. Eur Neuropsychopharmacol 26(5):828–840, 2016 26774661

Gordon OM, Salkovskis PM, Oldfield VB, et al: The association between obsessive compulsive disorder and obsessive compulsive personality disorder: prevalence and clinical presentation. Br J Clin Psychol 52(3):300–315, 2013 23865406

Grant BF, Stinson FS, Dawson DA, et al: Co-occurrence of 12-month alcohol and drug use disorders and personality disorders in the United States: results from the National Epidemiologic Survey on Alcohol and Related Conditions. Arch Gen Psychiatry 61(4):361–368, 2004 15066894

Grant JE: Co-occurrence of personality disorders in persons with kleptomania: a preliminary investigation. J Am Acad Psychiatry Law 32(4):395–398, 2004 15704625

Grant JE, Chamberlain SR: Impulsive action and impulsive choice across substance and behavioral addictions: cause or consequence? Addict Behav 39(11):1632–1639, 2014 24864028

Grant JE, Flynn M, Odlaug BL, et al: Personality disorders in gay, lesbian, bisexual, and transgender chemically dependent patients. Am J Addict 20(5):405–411, 2011 21838838

Grant JE, Mooney ME, Kushner MG: Prevalence, correlates, and comorbidity of DSM-IV obsessive-compulsive personality disorder: results from the National Epidemiologic Survey on Alcohol and Related Conditions. J Psychiatr Res 46(4):469–475, 2012 22257387

Hodgins DC, Stea JN, Grant JE: Gambling disorders. Lancet 378(9806):1874–1884, 2011 21600645

Irastorza Eguskiza LJ, Bellón JM, et al: Comorbidity of personality disorders and attention-deficit hyperactivity disorder in adults. Rev Psiquiatr Salud Ment 11(3):151–155, 2018 26968498

Jefferies K, Laws K, Fineberg NA: Cognitive and perceptual processing in body dysmorphic disorder. Eur Neuropsychopharmacol 20(Suppl 3):S309–S310, 2010

Laibson D: Golden eggs and hyperbolic discounting. Q J Econ 112(2):443–478, 1997

Lochner C, Simeon D, Niehaus DJ, et al: Trichotillomania and skin-picking: a phenomenological comparison. Depress Anxiety 15(2):83–86, 2002 11891999

Lochner C, Serebro P, van der Merwe L, et al: Comorbid obsessive-compulsive personality disorder in obsessive-compulsive disorder (OCD): a marker of severity. Prog Neuropsychopharmacol Biol Psychiatry 35(4):1087–1092, 2011 21411045

Logan GD, Cowan WB, Davis KA: On the ability to inhibit simple and choice reaction time responses: a model and a method. J Exp Psychol Hum Percept Perform 10(2):276–291, 1984 6232345

MacKillop J, Weafer J, C Gray J, et al: The latent structure of impulsivity: impulsive choice, impulsive action, and impulsive personality traits. Psychopharmacology (Berl) 233(18):3361–3370, 2016 27449350

Malloy-Diniz L, Fuentes D, Leite WB, et al: Impulsive behavior in adults with attention deficit/hyperactivity disorder: characterization of attentional, motor and cognitive impulsiveness. J Int Neuropsychol Soc 13(4):693–698, 2007 17521490

Mancebo MC, Eisen JL, Grant JE, et al: Obsessive compulsive personality disorder and obsessive compulsive disorder: clinical characteristics, diagnostic difficulties, and treatment. Ann Clin Psychiatry 17(4):197–204, 2005 16402751

Melca IA, Yücel M, Mendlowicz MV, et al: The correlates of obsessive-compulsive, schizotypal, and borderline personality disorders in obsessive-compulsive disorder. J Anxiety Disord 33:15–24, 2015 25956558

Neziroglu F, Rabinowitz D, Breytman A, et al: Skin picking phenomenology and severity comparison. Prim Care Companion J Clin Psychiatry 10(4):306–312, 2008 18787665

Patton JH, Stanford MS, Barratt ES: Factor structure of the Barratt Impulsiveness Scale. J Clin Psychol 51(6):768–774, 1995 8778124

Peters J, Büchel C: The neural mechanisms of inter-temporal decision-making: understanding variability. Trends Cogn Sci 15(5):227–239, 2011 21497544

Petry NM, Stinson FS, Grant BF: Comorbidity of DSM-IV pathological gambling and other psychiatric disorders: results from the National Epidemiologic Survey on Alcohol and Related Conditions. J Clin Psychiatry 66(5):564–574, 2005 15889941

Pinto A, Steinglass JE, Greene AL, et al: Capacity to delay reward differentiates obsessive-compulsive disorder and obsessive-compulsive personality disorder. Biol Psychiatry 75(8):653–659, 2014 24199665

Raymond NC, Coleman E, Miner MH: Psychiatric comorbidity and compulsive/impulsive traits in compulsive sexual behavior. Compr Psychiatry 44(5):370–380, 2003 14505297

Roberts ME, Tchanturia K, Treasure JL: Exploring the neurocognitive signature of poor set-shifting in anorexia and bulimia nervosa. J Psychiatr Res 44(14):964–970, 2010 20398910

Rogers RD, Everitt BJ, Baldacchino A, et al: Dissociable deficits in the decision-making cognition of chronic amphetamine abusers, opiate abusers, patients with focal damage to prefrontal cortex, and tryptophan-depleted normal volunteers: evidence for monoaminergic mechanisms. Neuropsychopharmacology 20(4):322–339, 1999 10088133

Samuels J, Nestadt G, Bienvenu OJ, et al: Personality disorders and normal personality dimensions in obsessive-compulsive disorder. Br J Psychiatry 177:457–462, 2000 11060001

Sansone RA, Hendricks CM, Sellbom M, et al: Anxiety symptoms and healthcare utilization among a sample of outpatients in an internal medicine clinic. Int J Psychiatry Med 33(2):133–139, 2003 12968826

Sansone RA, Hendricks CM, Gaither GA, et al: Prevalence of anxiety symptoms among a sample of outpatients in an internal medicine clinic: a pilot study. Depress Anxiety 19(2):133–136, 2004 15022149

Schlosser S, Black DW, Blum N, et al: The demography, phenomenology, and family history of 22 persons with compulsive hair pulling. Ann Clin Psychiatry 6(3):147–152, 1994a 7881494

Schlosser S, Black DW, Repertinger S, et al: Compulsive buying: demography, phenomenology, and comorbidity in 46 subjects. Gen Hosp Psychiatry 16(3):205–212, 1994b 8063088

Sica C, Bottesi G, Orsucci A, et al: "Not just right experiences" are specific to obsessive-compulsive disorder: further evidence from Italian clinical samples. J Anxiety Disord 31:73–83, 2015 25743760

Stanford MS, Mathias CW, Dougherty DM, et al: Fifty years of the Barratt Impulsiveness Scale: an update and review. Pers Individ Dif 47(5):385–395, 2009

Starcevic V, Berle D, Brakoulias V, et al: Obsessive-compulsive personality disorder co-occurring with obsessive-compulsive disorder: conceptual and clinical implications. Aust N Z J Psychiatry 47(1):65–73, 2013 22689335

Stein DJ, Hollander E: Obsessive-compulsive spectrum disorders. J Clin Psychiatry 56(6):265–266, 1995 7775369

van den Heuvel OA, van Wingen G, Soriano-Mas C, et al: Brain circuitry of compulsivity. Eur Neuropsychopharmacol 26(5):810–827, 2016 26711687

Villemarette-Pittman NR, Stanford MS, Greve KW, et al: Obsessive-compulsive personality disorder and behavioral disinhibition. J Psychol 138(1):5–22, 2004 15098711

Whitton AE, Henry JD, Grisham JR: Moral rigidity in obsessive-compulsive disorder: do abnormalities in inhibitory control, cognitive flexibility and disgust play a role? J Behav Ther Exp Psychiatry 45(1):152–159, 2014 24161700

Zadra S, Bischof G, Besser B, et al: The association between Internet addiction and personality disorders in a general population-based sample. J Behav Addict 5(4):691–699, 2016 28005417

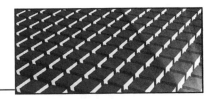

CHAPTER 6

OCPD AND AGGRESSION

Emil F. Coccaro, M.D.

Case Vignette

Frances is a 30-year-old female who lives with her boyfriend. She was raised in a "very strict" sect of Protestantism and currently continues to go to church regularly. After her parents divorced when she was 3 years old, she was raised primarily by her grandparents. Despite this, she saw her mother one to three times a month and saw her father every other weekend. She denied any knowledge of her father having emotional problems but did report that her mother "must have had emotional problems" because her mother left her when Frances was 10 years old. Frances denied history of physical or sexual abuse while growing up.

Frances's first reported mental health contact was at age 22 when she was having problems with her work supervisor because of her anger issues and work performance. Detailed psychiatric history revealed a single episode of major depression, now in full remission, that resolved within 6 months when she was 22 years old. In addition, she indicated that she has had frequent aggressive outbursts since age 10. These outbursts involve heated arguments, breaking things in her sight, and physical assaults. For example, during a chaotic time at work, Frances

99

was asked to transfer an employee under her supervision to another department in the store. She was upset at this challenge to her authority and sense of order, and in response, she yelled and screamed insults at her direct supervisor. As a result, she was suspended for a day. Another time, she got into a verbal fight with a coworker for "not obeying the rules" at work and slammed a glass vase on the coworker's desk, breaking the vase into many pieces. Her coworker was too afraid to report this incident to the supervisor. As a final example, Frances reported that she started an argument with her boyfriend because he hadn't paid the heating bill on time. She pushed him and hit him, causing bruises on his arms. Her boyfriend left her for a few weeks, although they eventually reconciled.

In addition to these dramatic behaviors, Frances also reports five of the DSM-5 criteria for OCPD (American Psychiatric Association 2013): 1) preoccupation with details (e.g., she reports that when preparing for a new hospital to open, she was so focused on filling secretarial roles that she failed to notice when someone was a good fit for another job and, thus, wasted time having to reinterview people later); 2) excessive devotion to work (she says that she works 12-hour days 5 days a week and that her family, boyfriend, boss, and coworkers all complain that she works too much); 3) inability to discard worthless objects (she reports being unable to throw out "tons of old papers and 15-year-old bills" because she might need them one day, something others have chided her for); 4) reluctance to delegate tasks (she reports doing a lot of jobs herself because she doesn't trust people to do them the "right way" and says that she has allowed her boyfriend to pay the bills only once in their 8-year relationship because she cannot trust he will do it in a timely manner); and 5) rigidity and stubbornness (she reports that she has these characteristics and that others describe her as being "set in her ways," to which she responds, "This is just the way I am").

As described previously in this volume, obsessive-compulsive personality disorder (OCPD) is a personality disorder characterized as having enduring and prominent traits of control, orderliness, perfectionism, stubbornness, rigidity, hoarding-like behavior, and indecisiveness. Its prevalence in the United States is about 8%, with similar prevalence rates in both sexes (Grant et al. 2012). Review of the basic features of OCPD does not suggest that such individuals should be at risk for aggressive tendencies and behavior, but recent studies focusing on aggression in individuals with personality disorders provide evidence that aggression is higher in individuals with OCPD than in those without it (Stein et al. 1996). In this chapter, we summarize data from studies in our research program in which we studied healthy volunteers without any lifetime psychiatric or personality disorder ($n=460$) and volunteers with any of a variety of mood, anxiety, and personality disorders ($n=1,182$). In this data set, 182 individuals (11.1%) met DSM-5 criteria for OCPD.

OCPD AND MEASURES OF AGGRESSION

Aggression is a multidimensional construct. Our research program focuses on two aspects of aggression: 1) aggression proneness (as measured by the Buss-Perry Aggression Questionnaire [BPAQ]; Buss and Perry 1992) and 2) actual aggressive behavior (as measured by the Life History of Aggression [LHA]; Coccaro et al. 1997). Analysis of data from our research program reveals that individuals with OCPD scored higher on the BPAQ (41.67±1.14 [95% confidence interval (CI): 39.44–43.91]) and the LHA (14.52±0.48 [95% CI: 13.58–15.45]) than do healthy control subjects (BPAQ: 28.10±0.69 [95% CI: 26.94–29.46]; LHA: 4.90±0.31 [95% CI: 4.29–5.52]). Closer analysis, however, reveals that a subgroup of OCPD individuals also met DSM-5 criteria for intermittent explosive disorder (IED), which may account for high aggression scores among those with OCPD. Reconfiguring the data to examine the effect of IED on OCPD revealed that individuals with OCPD still had higher BPAQ and LHA scores than did healthy control volunteers but not significantly higher aggression scores than others with psychiatric and/or personality disorder without IED (Figure 6–1). This means that, in the absence of meeting criteria for IED, individuals with OCPD are more aggressive than healthy control subjects only because aggression scores also run higher in those with psychopathology. In fact, aggression scores of those with OCPD and IED did not differ from scores of those with IED alone, suggesting that it is the pathology of IED that accounts for higher aggression scores among individuals with OCPD.

OCPD AND MEASURES OF IMPULSIVITY

Like aggression, impulsivity can also be assessed in terms of impulsivity proneness (as measured by the Barratt Impulsiveness Scale [BIS]; Patton et al. 1995) and actual impulsive behavior (as measured by the Life History of Impulsive Behavior [LHIB]; Coccaro and Schmidt-Kaplan 2012). In data from our research program, individuals with OCPD scored higher on the BIS than healthy control (HC) subjects (55.52±0.62); the scores for individuals with OCPD were similar to those for individuals with psychiatric and/or personality disorder but without OCPD (PC) (66.2±0.45). In contrast, individuals with OCPD had the highest scores on LHIB (OCPD: 57.07±2.72 vs. HC: 23.05±1.55 vs. PC: 47.20±1.13).

Because impulsivity is also characteristic of individuals with IED, we repeated the analysis without individuals who met criteria for IED (Figure 6–1). These analyses revealed that individuals with OCPD alone (i.e., without IED) are more impulsive than healthy control subjects but not more impulsive than those with psychiatric and/or per-

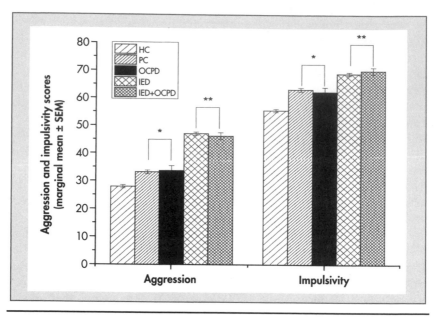

FIGURE 6–1.   Marginal means (±standard error of the mean) after analysis of covariance (age, sex, ethnicity, socioeconomic status as covariates) for Buss-Perry Aggression Questionnaire (BPAQ) Aggression and Barratt Impulsiveness Scale (BIS) Impulsivity scores.

Note.   HC=healthy control subjects; IED=participants with intermittent explosive disorder; OCPD=participants with obsessive-compulsive personality disorder; PC=psychiatric control subjects without OCPD. Single asterisks represent $p<0.05$; double asterisks represent $p<0.01$.

sonality disorder without OCPD; those with both OCPD and IED were more impulsive than the remaining groups. Accordingly, although individuals with OCPD are more impulsive than healthy control subjects, they are significantly less impulsive than those with both OCPD and IED, indicating that the addition of substantial aggressive proneness and behavior (in IED) enhances the presence of impulsivity.

BIOLOGICAL FEATURES OF OCPD WITH AND WITHOUT AGGRESSION

Serotonin

Over the years, we have examined the relationship of aggression with a variety of biomarkers. For serotonin (5-HT), these have included pharmacological challenge studies of the serotonin system with *d*-fenfluramine (d-FEN; Coccaro et al. 2010a) and the binding of tritiated paroxetine (^{3}H-PAROX; Coccaro et al. 2010b) to circulating platelets to quantify the number of 5-HT transporter (5-HTT) binding sites. The prolactin response to d-FEN (PRL[d-FEN]) has been reported to be low in individuals with IED and to correlate inversely with psychometric measures of aggression (Coccaro et al. 2010a). The same can be said of the platelet binding of ^{3}H-PAROX (Coccaro et al. 2010b). In our studies with PRL[d-FEN] response, we found that individuals with OCPD (without IED) have PRL[d-FEN] responses similar to those of individuals with IED, although individuals with IED alone have PRL[d-FEN] responses that are significantly lower than those of healthy control subjects (Figure 6–2). For the platelet ^{3}H-PAROX, individuals with OCPD±IED (1,365±170) were midway between individuals with IED alone (1,231±75) and those with OCPD alone (1,487±147), although none of these differences reached statistical significance.

Inflammatory Proteins

Human aggressive behavior also correlates with plasma levels of inflammatory proteins such as C-reactive protein (CRP; Coccaro 2006; Coccaro et al. 2014; Marsland et al. 2008), soluble interleukin-1 receptor-II (sIL-1RII; Coccaro et al. 2016b), and interleukin-6 (IL-6; Coccaro et al. 2014; Marsland et al. 2008; Suarez 2003). In addition, circulating levels of these inflammatory proteins are elevated in individuals with IED compared with healthy and psychiatric control subjects (Coccaro et al. 2014). When comparing a composite of these inflammatory proteins as a function of IED and OCPD, we see that individuals with OCPD alone have similar levels of these inflammatory proteins compared with healthy and psychiatric controls; it is only among individuals with IED and those with IED±OCPD that we see elevated plasma levels of these inflammatory proteins (Figure 6–2).

Neuroimaging

Our studies involving neuroimaging found that aggressive individuals have lower gray matter volume in frontolimbic circuits, including the orbitofrontal cortex, medial-prefrontal cortex, anterior cingulate cortex, amygdala, insula, and uncus (Coccaro et al. 2016a). Analyzing our volumetric-based morphometry data, we found that gray matter volume in individuals with OCPD (0.57± 0.02) did not differ from that in healthy control subjects (0.56±0.01), psychiatric control subjects (0.55±0.01), or even individuals with IED alone (0.52±0.01) but were significantly higher than in individuals with OCPD and IED (0.50±0.01), suggesting that the comorbidity of the two may account for

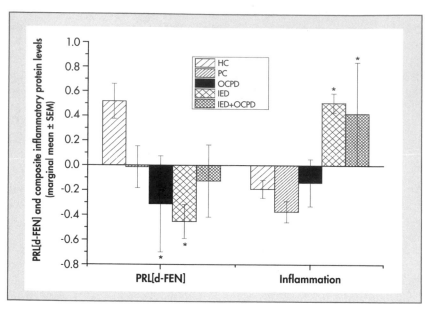

FIGURE 6–2.   Marginal means (±standard error of the mean) after analysis of covariance (age, sex, ethnicity, socioeconomic status as covariates) for PRL[d-FEN] residual (see Coccaro et al. 2010a) and composite (see text) inflammatory markers.

Note.   HC=healthy controls; IED=participants with intermittent explosive disorder; OCPD=participants with obsessive-compulsive personality disorder; PC=controls with psychiatric and/or personality disorder but without OCPD; PRL[d-FEN]=prolactin response to d-FEN. The asterisk represents $p<0.05$.

a greater loss of gray matter volume than IED alone. Reanalysis of functional neuroimaging studies using a social threat paradigm in a functional magnetic resonance imaging (fMRI) setting revealed that the amygdala response to social threat (anger faces) is much higher in individuals with IED alone (0.33 ± 0.06 arbitrary units) than in healthy control subjects (0.07 ± 0.06 arbitrary units). Although the difference in individuals with both IED and OCPD (0.07 ± 0.12 arbitrary units) was not significantly different from that in individuals with IED alone, this was likely due to the small number of individuals with OCPD and IED. From these two studies, it would appear that the presence of OCPD by itself, without comorbid IED, does not impact frontolimbic gray matter or the amygdala response to social threat as does the presence of IED.

TREATMENT CONSIDERATIONS

Given the findings discussed in the previous section, it is clear that impulsive aggressiveness (in IED) can be comorbid with OCPD even though the diagnostic criteria of OCPD do not include behaviors that are directly related to aggression. That said, we have found that the co-occurrence of the two disorders is far from rare. Because no community surveys have assessed both OCPD and IED, we can estimate the degree of comorbidity of the two only from our own clinical research studies of IED and mood, anxiety, and personality disorders. In our studies we found a significantly elevated risk of OCPD in individuals with IED (17.5% rate in IED vs. 5.5% rate in control subjects; odds ratio: 3.48 [95% CI: 2.50–4.86]; Coccaro et al. 2018). Not only is this statistically significant, but population prevalence estimates for IED (3.8%) and OCPD (8.0%) put the comorbidity risk at only about 0.3% if due to chance alone. Thus, this comorbidity represents more than a result of chance.

Although IED is also comorbid with a number of other disorders, especially personality disorders such as antisocial, borderline, narcissistic, and paranoid personality disorders (Coccaro et al. 2018), OCPD has significant comorbidity even in the presence of these other personality disorders, albeit lower than when examined alone (odds ratio: 2.42 [95% CI: 1.63–3.58]). Drilling down to the symptom level, the rigidity and stubbornness of OCPD are what account for the comorbidity of OCPD with IED (odds ratio: 2.79 [95% CI: 1.71–4.55]). Thus, it is not surprising that pharmacological treatment studies of aggression recruit individuals with IED and OCPD. Across our pharmacological treatment trials of aggression, we recruited participants with the following primary personality disorders: borderline (26.4%), antisocial (22.4%), obsessive-compulsive (20.9%), paranoid (19.4%), and narcissistic (13.8%), and then the remaining five personality disorders, with percentages ranging from 0.5 (schizotypal personality disorder) to 7.1% (avoidant personality disorder). Notably, we found no evidence that the antiaggressive response to a 5-HT agent (i.e., fluoxetine) in individuals with IED and OCPD is any different from the response in individuals with IED but without OCPD.

CASE VIGNETTE DISCUSSION

As described at the beginning of this chapter, Frances has both OCPD and IED. Traits of OCPD have been present since her adolescence, if not earlier, and so has her impulsive aggressive behavior. Her risk for OCPD was heightened during her childhood when she was split from her parents at age 3 years to live with her grandparents. Although she reports they were reasonably good to her, she also reports that she never really felt safe and was always hoping for her parents to come back. Not only did her parents not reunite, but when Frances was 10 years old, her mother disappeared from her life completely. This stressful life event solidified her feeling of not being in control of her environment and also set her up for emotional dysregulation and difficulty controlling her anger. Her impulsive, angry, aggressive outbursts are typically triggered by a challenge to her sense of order and her need to keep things under control. Although these traits may be treated with psychotherapy, Frances has come for treatment of her anger issues because these issues prompted her boyfriend to move out for a few weeks. Her aggressiveness can be treated with cognitive-behavioral therapy and/or medication. After her initial evaluation, Frances opted for a trial of a serotonergic selective agent (fluoxetine). She started taking 20 mg/day, and the dosage was increased to 40 mg/day after 4 weeks. She experienced no lasting side effects and she began to report many fewer impulsive aggressive outbursts within 2 months of beginning the medication. She has continued to do well and is now in psychodynamic therapy working on issues related to her OCPD.

TAKE-HOME POINTS

- Individuals with OCPD are more aggressive and impulsive than healthy control subjects but not more aggressive than control subjects with nonaggressive psychiatric and/or personality disorders. They are also less aggressive than those with a primary impulsive aggressive disorder (i.e., IED).

- When it comes to biological features that are abnormal in individuals with a primary impulsive aggression disorder (e.g., number of 5-HTT binding sites, plasma levels of inflammatory proteins), individuals with OCPD without a comorbid impulsive aggression disorder look like control subjects who have other nonaggressive psychiatric or personality disorders.

- The antiaggressive response to fluoxetine of individuals with OCPD and a comorbid impulsive aggression disorder does not differ from the response of individuals who have other personality disorders and comorbid impulsive aggression. Impulsive aggression in individuals with OCPD may be treated in the same fashion as in those with other comorbid disorders with impulsive aggressive behavior.

REFERENCES

American Psychiatric Association: Diagnostic and Statistical Manual of Mental Disorders, 5th Edition. Arlington, VA, American Psychiatric Association, 2013

Buss AH, Perry M: The Aggression Questionnaire. J Pers Soc Psychol 63(3):452–459, 1992 1403624

Coccaro EF: Association of C-reactive protein elevation with trait aggression and hostility in personality disordered subjects: a pilot study. J Psychiatr Res 40(5):460–465, 2006 15993896

Coccaro EF, Schmidt-Kaplan CA: Life history of impulsive behavior: development and validation of a new questionnaire. J Psychiatr Res 46(3):346–352, 2012 22212770

Coccaro EF, Berman ME, Kavoussi RJ: Assessment of life history of aggression: development and psychometric characteristics. Psychiatry Res 73(3):147–157, 1997 9481806

Coccaro EF, Lee R, Kavoussi RJ: Aggression, suicidality, and intermittent explosive disorder: serotonergic correlates in personality disorder and healthy control subjects. Neuropsychopharmacology 35(2):435–444, 2010a 19776731

Coccaro EF, Lee R, Kavoussi RJ: Inverse relationship between numbers of 5-HT transporter binding sites and life history of aggression and intermittent explosive disorder. J Psychiatr Res 44(3):137–142, 2010b 19767013

Coccaro EF, Lee R, Coussons-Read M: Elevated plasma inflammatory markers in individuals with intermittent explosive disorder and correlation with aggression in humans. JAMA Psychiatry 71(2):158–165, 2014 24352431

Coccaro EF, Fitzgerald DA, Lee R, et al: Frontolimbic morphometric abnormalities in intermittent explosive disorder and aggression. Biol Psychiatry Cogn Neurosci Neuroimaging 1(1):32–38, 2016a 29560894

Coccaro EF, Lee R, Fanning JR, et al: Tryptophan, kynurenine, and kynurenine metabolites: relationship to lifetime aggression and inflammatory markers in human subjects. Psychoneuroendocrinology 71:189–196, 2016b 27318828

Coccaro EF, Shima CK, Lee RJ: Comorbidity of personality disorder with intermittent explosive disorder. J Psychiatr Res 106:15–21, 2018 30240963

Grant JE, Mooney ME, Kushner MG: Prevalence, correlates, and comorbidity of DSM-IV obsessive-compulsive personality disorder: results from the National Epidemiologic Survey on Alcohol and Related Conditions. J Psychiatr Res 46(4):469–475, 2012 22257387

Marsland AL, Prather AA, Petersen KL, et al: Antagonistic characteristics are positively associated with inflammatory markers independently of trait negative emotionality. Brain Behav Immun 22(5):753–761, 2008 18226879

Patton JH, Stanford MS, Barratt ES: Factor structure of the Barratt Impulsiveness Scale. J Clin Psychol 51(6):768–774, 1995 8778124

Stein DJ, Trestman RL, Mitropoulou V, et al: Impulsivity and serotonergic function in compulsive personality disorder. J Neuropsychiatry Clin Neurosci 8(4):393–398, 1996 9116474

Suarez EC: Joint effect of hostility and severity of depressive symptoms on plasma interleukin-6 concentration. Psychosom Med 65(4):523–527, 2003 12883100

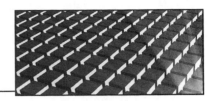

CHAPTER 7

GENDER AND CULTURAL ASPECTS OF OCPD

Leonardo F. Fontenelle, M.D., Ph.D.

Julliana N. Quintas, M.D.

Lucy Albertella, Ph.D.

CASE VIGNETTES

Case 1

Alec, a 35-year-old wealthy and successful engineer working in a transnational company, sought treatment because of marital problems related to his excessive need for control of his wife's behaviors and schedule. He reported persistent sadness, anhedonia, neurovegetative symptoms, and thoughts of suicide. His psychiatrist diagnosed a major depressive episode but never considered a diagnosis of obsessive-compulsive personality disorder (OCPD).

Case 2

Britney, a 25-year-old sales assistant, sought treatment for being unable to delegate tasks to her coworkers unless they followed exactly her way of doing things, as well as several other symptoms that are common in OCPD. However, Britney was reluctant to agree to a diagnosis of and treatment for OCPD, particularly because she heard from her family members that her overzealousness with money was not a symptom but rather a feature of her Scottish background.

Case 3

Kristoff, an 80-year-old Scandinavian retiree who immigrated to Rio de Janeiro in the 1940s, was referred to a neurobehavioral clinic for the assessment of memory complaints. Although no consistent cognitive deficits emerged, a diagnosis of OCPD was entertained, partly because of Kristoff's preoccupation with details, lack of interpersonal warmth, and complaints about his inability to express affection to Latin American family members.

Case 4

Dan, a 40-year-old farmer, sought treatment in our clinic for a pervasive pattern of inflexibility and stubbornness. After being successfully treated for OCPD, he was referred to a general practitioner, who eventually disagreed with the diagnosis, withdrew Dan's medications, and argued that Dan's preoccupation with rules and deference to authority figures reflected the fact that he was raised in a traditional Japanese family.

Gender and culture are recognized to play a significant role in psychopathology. They are known to aggravate, attenuate, and shape different expressions of mental distress. For instance, with regard to obsessive-compulsive disorder (OCD), a condition at the center of the category of obsessive-compulsive and related disorders that was introduced in DSM-5 (American Psychiatric Association 2013), males are known to display an earlier onset and more severe clinical picture, and individuals hailing from the Middle East tend to exhibit more religious concerns (Fontenelle et al. 2004). It is beyond the scope of this chapter to address the influence of gender and culture on psychopathology more broadly, but rather, the aim of this chapter is to provide an overview of their impact on personality, particularly in OCPD. To this end, an initial word of caution is needed: the impact of gender and cultural factors on personality is a sensitive issue because stereotypes always have the potential to confound true clinical variations between people of different genders and cultures with pseudoscientific observations and/or mere superficial remarks made by unskilled clinicians who are unable to establish rapport with their patients (Chess et al. 1953).

DEFINITIONS

Understanding of the roles that gender and culture play with regard to psychopathology requires a close collaboration between clinicians and colleagues from the human sciences, who can provide precise definitions for a more detailed analysis of this topic (West and Zimmerman 1987). Unfortunately, the literature on personality disorders has frequently employed the terms *sex* and *gender* interchangeably, despite their different meanings (Eaton and Greene 2018; Schulte Holthausen and Habel 2018). It is now agreed that *sex* is a determination made through the application of biological criteria (e.g., genitalia or chromosomal type) for classifying persons as females or males (West and Zimmerman 1987). By contrast, *gender* is now widely recognized as "the lived role as boy or girl, man or woman" (American Psychiatric Association 2013, p. 451). On the basis of these differences and on the ever-increasing importance of gender-related issues in modern societies, a recent review has recommended that researchers on sex and gender correlates of psychopathology use the following terms (Hartung and Lefler 2019):

- *Cisgender females:* biological females who identify as female
- *Cisgender males:* biological males who identify as male
- *Noncisgender females:* transgender females or intersex individuals who identify as female
- *Noncisgender males:* transgender males or intersex individuals who identify as male
- *Nonbinary/gender-queer:* individuals who do not subscribe to a binary gender identity

Alternatively, researchers and clinicians can employ scales to assess gender roles (masculinity vs. femininity) (Kachel et al. 2016).

DSM-5 considers cultural formulation and includes useful definitions for culture, ethnicity, and race. According to DSM-5, *"culture* refers to systems of knowledge, concepts, rules, and practices that are learned and transmitted across generations" (American Psychiatric Association 2013, p. 749). Cultures have been described as fluid systems that undergo continuous change over time. In a globalized society, most individuals are exposed to multiple cultures, which may help shape their identities to different extents. Another concept that is relevant for our discussion is *ethnicity*, defined as a "culturally constructed group identity used to define peoples and communities" (American Psychiatric Association 2013, p. 749). Ethnicity can be based on different factors, including history, geography, language, religion, or other characteristics that distinguish one group from others. Finally, DSM-5 defines *race* as a "culturally constructed category of identity that divides humanity into groups based on a variety of superficial physical traits attributed to some hypothetical intrinsic, biological characteristics" (American Psychiatric Association 2013, p. 749). Importantly, the concept of race has no clear biological meaning, but it is important from a social perspective because it has supported racism, discrimination, and social exclusion, all of which can have strong negative effects on mental health.

APPROACHES TO GENDER AND CULTURE IN DSM-IV AND DSM-5

Since DSM-IV, the roles played by sex/gender and culture in the presentation, assessment, treatment, and outcome of mental disorders have been given extra attention (American Psychiatric Association 2000). In DSM-IV this importance is noted 1) in the main text, through a discussion of specific culture, age, and gender features relevant for the clinical presentations of disorders, and 2) in an appendix that includes both a glossary of culture-bound syndromes and an outline for cultural formulation designed to assist the clinician in systematically evaluating and reporting the impact of the individual's cultural context (American Psychiatric Association 2000). In DSM-5, this outline has been removed from the appendix and included in a new Section III, "Emerging Measures and Models," which attests to the increased emphasis given to cultural aspects of mental disorders in the current edition of the manual. This new section also includes the Cultural Formulation Interview (CFI), which has been field tested for diagnostic usefulness among clinicians and for acceptability among patients (American Psychiatric Association 2013). According to DSM-5, the CFI may be particularly useful in the presence of culturally related difficulties relating to 1) the diagnostic process, 2) the fit between culturally distinctive symptoms and DSM-5 criteria, 3) the assessment of impairment or severity of illness, 4) reaching a consensus between the clinician and the individual regarding the course of care, or 5) engagement in or adherence to treatment.

GENDER

Gender and Personality

In the seminal meta-analysis by Feingold (1994), spanning more than 50 years of research on personality, males were found to be more assertive and to have slightly higher self-esteem than females, who were higher in extroversion, anxiety, trust, and tender-mindedness (e.g., nurturance). This meta-analysis did not find remarkable differences in social anxiety, impulsiveness, activity, ideas (e.g., reflectiveness), locus of control, and orderliness. Of note, the identified differences were constant across ages, years of data collection, educational levels, and nations.

More recently, a study using the five-factor model (FFM), which includes extroversion, agreeableness, neuroticism, conscientiousness, and openness/intellect domains, found women to exhibit greater total scores on extroversion, agreeableness, and neuroticism (Weisberg et al. 2011). In contrast, differences between genders in terms of conscientiousness and openness/intellect were restricted to the subdomain levels—that is, women (particularly at younger ages) scored higher on orderliness and lower on industriousness, whereas men scored lower on openness and higher on intellect (Weisberg et al. 2011). Curiously, one study (Borkenau et al. 2013) found that people tend to provide more varied accounts of personality of males than of females, with females giving more varied descriptions than do males. Of note, these effects were stronger in more individualistic societies.

Feingold (1994) also reviewed a number of theories that have been put forward to explain differences between sexes/genders in terms of personality, including biological (i.e., temperamental) accounts or sociocultural models. In terms of sociocultural models, at least three social theories exist to explain sex/gender dimorphism: 1) the social role model, which suggests that social behaviors stem from gender roles that dictate behaviors that are appropriate for males and females; 2) the expectancy model, which suggests that holders of stereotypical beliefs treat others in ways that lead others to conform to the prejudices of the perceivers; and 3) the artifact model, according to which differences stem from the importance that people from different sexes/genders give to having certain traits, thus affecting self-report responses. Feingold argued that biological and sociocultural reasons are not mutually exclusive and may influence particular moments in the lives of human beings—that is, biological factors are innate and therefore more likely to exert more proximal or early influences, whereas sociocultural factors play a greater role distally or later in life. However, Feingold failed to mention a number of biological factors that have a potential to shape personality traits later in life, such as exposure to hormones during puberty (Schutter et al. 2017).

Gender and Personality Disorders

The literature consistently shows differences in the prevalence of most "classic" DSM personality disorders across different sexes/genders. A recent review (Schulte Holthausen and Habel 2018) showed that schizoid, schizotypal, antisocial, narcissistic, and obsessive-compulsive personality disorders were more commonly reported in males, whereas borderline, histrionic, and dependent personality disorders were more frequently diagnosed in females.

In DSM-5, an alternative hybrid personality model including the domains of negative affectivity, detachment, antagonism, disinhibition, and psychoticism (based on the FFM-related concepts of neuroticism, extroversion, agreeableness, conscientiousness, and openness, respectively) has been proposed, also with potential relevance for the study of the impact of sex/gender in personality disorders (American Psychiatric Association 2013; Oltmanns and Powers 2012). According to this new model, personality disorders are perceived as combinations of otherwise "normal" traits that are inflexible, pervasive, and stable and that also result in impaired functioning (Oltmanns and Powers 2012). Studies of the FFM show that women score higher on negative affectivity and lower on antagonism (Costa et al. 2001; Feingold 1994; Schmitt et al. 2008)—findings that are consistent with borderline and dependent personality disorders being more prevalent among females (Oltmanns and Powers 2012). In contrast, lower levels of negative affectivity and greater levels of antagonism in men (Chapman et al. 2007; Feingold 1994) dovetail with studies showing antisocial personality disorder to be more prevalent among males (Oltmanns and Powers 2012).

A few authors have argued that the diagnostic criteria for personality disorders, or the ways in which clinicians and researchers use the diagnostic manuals, may bias the diagnosis of these disorders toward a given gender (i.e., the so-called criterion bias or assessment bias, respectively) (Oltmanns and Powers 2012). Oltmanns and Powers contended that these biases also have unwanted consequences in terms of prevalence rates across sexes/genders. For instance, they suggested that women are more likely to be diagnosed with a dependent personality disorder because that condition is based on feminine traits (e.g., putting the needs of others ahead of one's own), which have also been labeled as maladaptive (Oltmanns and Powers 2012). Thus, these definitions have transformed gender into "disorders" at the cost of minimizing women's attempts to cope with an oppressive society (Oltmanns and Powers 2012). However, whether these theoretical fragilities represent a threat to the validity of personality disorder constructs or to differences in their prevalence across sexes/genders is questionable. Other traits typically considered masculine (e.g., difficulty in expressing emotions, workaholism) not only are part of a few personality disorders (e.g., schizotypal personality disorder and OCPD) but also are listed as potentially maladaptive (Oltmanns and Powers 2012).

Gender and OCPD

Despite the clinical and epidemiological importance of OCPD, which has repeatedly been reported as the most common personality disorder in treatment-seeking and non-treatment-seeking settings (see Chapter 2, "Diagnosis and Clinical Features of OCPD"), the literature on the impact of sex/gender in OCPD remains sparse. The few existing studies have compared male and female individuals with OCPD in terms of symptom expression (Cain et al. 2015), sociodemographic features (Grant et al. 2012), comorbidity patterns (Grant et al. 2012; Nestadt et al. 2009; Reas et al. 2013), and underlying neurobiology (Blom et al. 2011; Kanehisa et al. 2017). Moreover, with a few exceptions (Grant et al. 2012), these investigations have frequently recruited a small number of subjects and included sex/gender comparisons as less important, subsidiary analyses. For instance, comparisons between the frequencies of DSM-5 criteria exhibited by males versus females with OCPD are lacking yet would be very informative. One study suggested that laypeople perceive OCPD symptoms as being "more pathological" in males (Sprock et al. 2001).

To the best of our knowledge, however, the only study that compared OCPD patients from different genders in terms of their symptom expression contrasted 16 female and 9 male participants on the Systemizing Quotient Scale–Short (SQ-Short), which assesses drives to analyze variables in a system or to derive the system's governing rules (Cain et al. 2015). Consistent with previous research using normative controls (Baron-Cohen et al. 2003), more men than women in the OCPD group reported systemizing. Accordingly, Cain and colleagues speculated that interpersonal control among OCPD males, in contrast to females, may be more related to deriving rules, analyzing, and making predictions about another's behavior, which is consistent with increased systemizing. The interpersonal behavior of women with OCPD did not correlate with any particular variable in the Cain study.

To date, the biggest study of OCPD addressed its sociodemographic and comorbidity correlates in 43,093 adults from the National Epidemiologic Survey on Alcohol and Related Conditions (Grant et al. 2012). This study found that the prevalence of OCPD was 8%, with no significantly different rates for men and women (in contrast to findings of the studies reviewed by Schulte Holthausen and Habel [2018], discussed above). In this study, an OCPD diagnosis was more frequently reported in females from the lowest income strata, females who were married or cohabitating, and females who did not graduate from high school, thus suggesting that OCPD symptoms may be more tolerated or socially acceptable in males from higher income strata, males who are single, and males who are high school graduates. Broadly speaking, in terms of comorbidity with OCPD, lifetime and 12-month prevalence rates of alcohol and drug use disorders and schizoid and antisocial personality disorders were greater in men, whereas rates of depressive and anxiety disorders and paranoid and avoidant personality disorders were higher in women (Grant et al. 2012). In contrast, the prevalence of OCPD was higher in females with alcohol and drug use disorders and in males with depressive and anxiety disorders (Grant et al. 2012). After controlling for sociodemographic variables and other psychiatric disorders, only associations of OCPD with alcohol abuse and current mood and anxiety disorders remained significant, although diminished in magnitude (Grant et al. 2012).

In a Norwegian study with 3,266 consecutive and first admissions, assessed for different eating disorders, Reas et al. (2013) assigned each participant to a specific DSM-IV Axis II group (avoidant, borderline, paranoid, dependent, or obsessive-compulsive personality disorder) according to a hierarchical system: in cases of comorbid personality disorders, Cluster A diagnoses had precedence over Clusters B and C, and Cluster B had hierarchical precedence over Cluster C. In this study, a significant association was found for the co-occurrence of anorexia nervosa and OCPD in females but not in males. Furthermore, women diagnosed with anorexia nervosa met a significantly higher number of diagnostic criteria for OCPD than did women without anorexia nervosa.

In another study using data from 700 participants with OCD, Nestadt et al. (2009) performed a multilevel latent class analysis based on comorbid disorders and found a three-class solution. One of the classes, the "OCD co-morbid affective-related class," was characterized as being predominantly female with a young age at onset, OCPD features, high scores on the "taboo" factor of OCD symptoms, and low conscientiousness. Although it was somewhat surprising to find OCPD traits and lower conscientiousness in the same class, Samuel and Widiger (2011) noted that most conscientiousness items in the instrument used to assess conscientiousness (i.e., the Revised NEO Personality Inventory items) are keyed in the direction of adaptive rather than maladaptive functioning (see also Chapter 12, "Positive Aspects of OCPD"). Taken together, these studies suggest that OCPD in females is related to the presence of mood and anxiety disorders (Grant et al. 2012), anorexia nervosa (Reas et al. 2013), and OCD (Nestadt et al. 2009).

One study found that males but not females with OCPD differed from control subjects by showing decreased sympathetic and parasympathetic reactivity, as evidenced by decreased levels of salivary amylase and cortisol levels in response to social stress (Kanehisa et al. 2017). A different study, in which 374 community individuals were assessed for personality disorders with the International Personality Disorder Examination and were genotyped for the serotonin transporter promoter polymorphism (5HTTLPR, a degenerate repeat polymorphic region in the SLC6A4 gene), found no relationship between OCPD and 5HTTLPR in unstratified analyses (Blom et al. 2011). However, the allele variants had opposite effects in male and female subjects with OCPD. Male carriers of the short (s) allele of the 5HTTLPR polymorphism had significantly lower OCPD trait scores, whereas female s allele carriers tended to have higher OCPD trait scores. More specifically, the long (l) allele was significantly associated with different OCPD traits in males, particularly perfectionism, reluctance to delegate, and scrupulosity, with all of the remaining traits (with the exception of devotion to work) showing trends in the same direction. In contrast, the same seven OCPD traits showed a trend to be associated with the s allele in women. These incipient findings suggest that dysfunction of stress response mechanisms and serotonergic neurotransmission may play a greater role in men with OCPD than in women. Curiously, previous studies also found that the s allele in females may increase an individual's susceptibility to depression under stressful life conditions (Blom et al. 2011).

CULTURE

Culture and Personality

Cross-cultural comparisons of personality traits face problems due to imprecise scale translations, response biases, and unfamiliarity with questionnaires in some cultures (Terracciano and McCrae 2006). In general, the study of culture and personality can be divided into the universality versus uniqueness approaches to traits (the so-called etic-emic distinction): the transportation of personality measures across cultures (the etic approach) and the identification of indigenous dimensions (the emic approach) (Church 2016). Under the *etic* approach (derived from the term phon*etic*—i.e., the study of *universal* sounds in all languages), researchers have tested and successfully demonstrated the cross-cultural factor replicability of the FFM in up to 50 cultures (McCrae et al. 2005). Curiously, studies of FFM across cultures have shown similar profiles between Australians and New Zealanders, Burkinabé and Batswana, Germans and Austrians, Americans and Canadians, and Hong Kong and Taiwan Chinese (Terracciano and McCrae 2006). However, cross-cultural studies found it particularly difficult to replicate the FFM in less educated or preliterate groups, such as the Mooré in Burkina Faso or forager-farmers in Bolivia (Church 2016). In contrast to the etic approach, the *emic* approach (from the term phon*emics*—i.e., the study of the unique or language-specific meanings associated with particular sounds) identifies culture-specific personality constructs evident in native languages and identified by cultural informants. The emic approach has allowed replication of the FFM in some, but not all (e.g., Hindi), cultures.

Another important issue in terms of the relationship between culture and personality involves the mediating roles of sex/gender (Costa et al. 2001; Schmitt et al. 2017) and socioeconomic status (Schmitt et al. 2017). As discussed in the earlier section on gender and personality, males and females show consistent differences in terms of personality traits across a range of instruments. Social role theorists have argued that these differences reflect merely perceived gender roles, gender social-ization, and sociostructural power differentials. Surprisingly, however, the available evidence suggests that these gender differences are con-spicuously larger in cultures with more egalitarian gender roles, gender socialization, and sociopolitical gender equity (Schmitt et al. 2017). Po-tential reasons for this amplification include the fact that in an egalitar-ian society, certain behaviors (e.g., kindness) are more likely to be described as personality traits (e.g., agreeableness) rather than societal norms. Given the different socioeconomic conditions of people living in first- versus third-world countries and the well-known impact of socio-economic status on personality, it would be interesting to assess how culture and socioeconomic status interact to generate specific personal-ity patterns.

Culture and Personality Disorder

The relationship between personality and culture, particularly in terms of Western versus non-Western comparisons, has provided interesting insights. Arguably, in Western cultures, the self is generally considered an "object" separate from the world, located in an inner compartment and comprising distinctive habits, emotions, behaviors, intentions, and conflicts (Mulder 2012). In contrast, selves in non-Western societies have been described as being more "sociocentric," with individuals describing feeling more connected to other persons and social institutions (Mulder 2012). Moreover, whereas in Western societies, disordered personalities tend to be perceived as medical conditions that warrant evidence-based treatments by psychiatrists or psychologists, in non-Western cultures, personality problems are most likely considered to be poor personal choices put into practice by an exercise of free will and are remediated by civil, familial, or spiritual measures (Mulder 2012).

Clearly, the delineations of concepts of normality and abnormality, including the existence of personality problems as an illness (or disor-der), have been calibrated in terms of Western norms (Mulder 2012). That said, it remains unclear whether differences in prevalence rates of different personality disorders across diverse cultures reflect, in part, a biological phenomenon (linked, for instance, to the specific genetic makeup of a specific ethnic group) or are simply an artifact of societies that more or less tolerate certain types of behaviors, thus decreasing or increasing caseness, respectively.

The developers of DSM-5 tried their best to make the diagnosis of personality disorders culture-free. A personality disorder is defined in DSM-5 as an "enduring pattern of inner experience and behavior that *deviates markedly from the expectations of the individual's culture*, is pervasive and inflexible, has an onset in adolescence or early adulthood, is stable over time, and leads to distress or impairment" (American Psychiatric Association 2013, p. 645; italics added). Similarly, in the alternative DSM-5 model for personality disorders, essential features of a personality disorder are "impairments in personality functioning and the individual's personality trait expression [that] are not better understood as normal for an individual's developmental stage or sociocultural environment" (American Psychiatric Association 2013, p. 761). DSM-5 also mentions that clinicians should not consider as personality disorders any "habits, customs, or interpersonal styles that are culturally sanctioned by the individual's reference group" (American Psychiatric Association 2013, p. 681).

Nevertheless, it seems that personality disorders (particularly antisocial personality disorder) are a pancultural phenomenon, although prevalence rates may vary (Mulder 2012). To date, the most compelling evidence suggests that personality disorders, particularly Cluster B personality disorders, are more prevalent in Western cultures and in white as compared with black individuals (McGilloway et al. 2010). The fact that the rates of antisocial personality disorder, and possibly other personality disorders, have been increasing suggests that social and cultural factors play a significant role in determining such prevalence rates (Paris 1998).

Still, it seems difficult to dissociate cultural influences from personality disorders. For instance, there is reasonable evidence that the *goodness-of-fit* or the *personality-culture clash* between an individual's personality style and his or her society is associated with self-reported psychological distress, with potential diagnosis consequences for personality disorders (Mulder 2012). The fact that immigration seems to be associated with increasing rates of personality disorders supports this hypothesis, as does the fact that shy and unsociable individuals in collectivistic countries (e.g., Korea) tend to show better social and emotional adjustment than individuals with similar characteristics in an individualistic country (e.g., Australia) (Kim et al. 2008). Additionally, in Korea, being socially withdrawn is seen as well behaved and easily accepted by peers (Chen and Stevenson 1995).

Much of the research on the impact of culture in personality disorders has considered the differences between collectivistic and individualistic cultures. For instance, in collectivistic cultures, group membership is a central aspect of identity, and valued personal traits reflect the goals of collectivism (Mulder 2012). Life satisfaction derives from successfully carrying out social roles and obligations. Restraint in emotional expression, in order to promote in-group harmony, is valued. In contrast, individualism supports open emotional expression and striving to attain personal goals, traits deemed potentially inappropriate in collectivistic cultures (Mulder 2012). It is unclear whether the differences between collectivistic and individualistic cultures are relevant for OCPD diagnosis.

Culture and OCPD

As indicated at the start of this chapter, studies of racial aspects of personality do not seem to be very useful for the practicing physician because of potential bias, because they may have been undertaken on a superficial basis (Braun et al. 2007), and/or because of potentially harmful consequences (for a relevant discussion of OCD, see Williams and Jahn 2017). Although the concept of ethnicity is probably more useful, both for research and for clinical practice, the fact that *race* and *ethnicity* have been used interchangeably makes existing studies difficult to interpret. For instance, in the National Epidemiologic Survey on Alcohol and Related Conditions described in the subsection "Gender and OCPD," OCPD was found to be significantly less common among Asians or Pacific Islanders and Hispanics relative to whites in the United States (Grant et al. 2004, 2012). These differences were also reported in the male and female subsamples separately, but in the male subsamples, blacks were also less likely than whites to have OCPD (Grant et al. 2012). This study also found increased rates of OCPD in the Northeast and South compared with the Midwest or the West. The fact that these relationships were not reported in a clinical sample is noteworthy (Chavira et al. 2003). Finally, in a study with a Hispanic outpatient sample, a two-factor solution—perfectionism and interpersonal rigidity—replicated findings reported in previous studies in samples of individuals with European ancestry (Ansell et al. 2010).

In an early review of OCPD, Pollak (1979, p. 226) argued that "[m]any of the OCPD traits (e.g., perseverance, industriousness, thriftiness, ambition, self-control, and so on), are highly regarded and rewarded within capitalistic, technological societies, serve to promote in their possessors feelings of self-worth and acceptability, and generally provide them with a foundation for emotional stability and relative resistance to stress." Forty years after Pollak's review, the impact of cultural factors in OCPD remains elusive and poorly studied. It is possible, however, to use the personality-culture clash hypothesis to make a number of predictions about the role of culture in DSM-5 OCPD. These predictions, which we briefly outline below, are based on the definition of OCPD in DSM-5 as a "pervasive pattern of preoccupation with orderliness, perfectionism, and mental and interpersonal control, at the expense of flexibility, openness, and efficiency, beginning by early adulthood and present in a variety of contexts" (American Psychiatric Association 2013, p. 678).

For instance, preoccupation with orderliness (including "details, rules, lists, order, organization, or schedules") or perfectionism (e.g., "strict standards") (American Psychiatric Association 2013, p. 678) seems to characterize first-world countries but not third-world countries. Thus, one can speculate that individuals high on such traits would be more likely to experience distress and therefore to be diagnosed with OCPD in the first-world countries. Similarly, excessive mental control exemplified by overconscientiousness, scrupulosity, and inflexibility about matters of morality, ethics, or values (American Psychiatric Association 2013) may be particularly prominent in strictly religious (e.g., Middle Eastern) countries, suggesting that individuals raised in these societies might be more likely to be diagnosed with OCPD in more secular societies. Individuals showing high interpersonal control traits for imposing their ways of doing things on others would be more likely to have this feature described as a symptom in societies that are less authoritarian, with more democratic values. A miserly spending style, where money is viewed as something to be hoarded for future catastrophes, seems to be more likely to be a characteristic of individuals who hail from less economically developed countries or societies characterized by political and economic instabilities (American Psychiatric Association 2013).

Other aspects of OCPD that do not represent criteria but are nevertheless included in the DSM-5 text for OCPD include the fact that individuals with OCPD may be preoccupied with "dominance-submission relationships and may display excessive deference to an authority they respect" (American Psychiatric Association 2013, p. 680). Although not representing core symptoms, these features can be part of the latent OCPD construct. Accordingly, one can speculate that Eastern cultures that typically emphasize hierarchy, such as respect for older individuals, would be more likely to exhibit lower prevalence rates of OCPD. Alternatively, individuals with OCPD who enter into the military may be less inclined to experience distress or dysfunction in this regard as compared with individuals with other personality disorders. The DSM-5 text also describes the highly controlled or stilted affection (as in "affective isolation" or "reaction formation" mechanisms of defenses, respectively) (Nemiah and Appel 1961) and the discomfort individuals with OCPD may show in the presence of others who are emotionally expressive (American Psychiatric Association 2013). Because collectivistic cultures seem to be less tolerant of deviance (e.g., demonstrate inflexibility) and tend to promote behavioral patterns characterized by inhibition and constriction of emotion (affect isolation), one can speculate that individuals hailing from Eastern cultures would be more likely to be diagnosed with OCPD in modern individualistic societies, which value flexibility and less secure social roles.

CASE VIGNETTE DISCUSSION

The case vignettes introduced at the beginning of this chapter illustrate how information on gender and culture may interfere positively or negatively with the appropriate diagnosis and/or management of individuals with OCPD. In Alec's case, the diagnosis of OCPD is missed in a wealthy and educated male because OCPD traits are often considered more socially acceptable in such individuals. Britney's case exemplifies how unfounded stereotypes and stigma can interfere negatively with the appropriate treatment adherence of an OCPD patient. In the subsequent cases, it is possible to note that clinicians can raise appropriate (Kristoff's case) or inappropriate (Dan's case) diagnostic questions based on consistent cultural differences.

TAKE-HOME POINTS

- Both sex/gender and culture/ethnicity represent neglected variables in OCPD studies.
- Research findings suggest that sex/gender can impact clinical expression, comorbidity findings, and neurobiological variables in OCPD.
- Although culture and ethnicity have not been well studied in OCPD, it is possible to make several testable predictions in terms of how these variables impact the condition.

REFERENCES

American Psychiatric Association: Diagnostic and Statistical Manual of Mental Disorders, 4th Edition, Text Revision. Washington, DC, American Psychiatric Association, 2000

American Psychiatric Association: Diagnostic and Statistical Manual of Mental Disorders, 5th Edition. Arlington, VA, American Psychiatric Association, 2013

Ansell EB, Pinto A, Crosby RD, et al: The prevalence and structure of obsessive-compulsive personality disorder in Hispanic psychiatric outpatients. J Behav Ther Exp Psychiatry 41(3):275–281, 2010 20227063

Baron-Cohen S, Richler J, Bisarya D, et al: The systemizing quotient: an investigation of adults with Asperger syndrome or high-functioning autism, and normal sex differences. Philos Trans R Soc Lond B Biol Sci 358(1430):361–374, 2003 12639333

Blom RM, Samuels JF, Riddle MA, et al: Association between a serotonin transporter promoter polymorphism (5HTTLPR) and personality disorder traits in a community sample. J Psychiatr Res 45(9):1153–1159, 2011 21450307

Borkenau P, McCrae RR, Terracciano A: Do men vary more than women in personality? A study in 51 cultures. J Res Pers 47(2):135–144, 2013 23559686

Braun L, Fausto-Sterling A, Fullwiley D, et al: Racial categories in medical practice: how useful are they? PLoS Med 4(9):e271, 2007 17896853

Cain NM, Ansell EB, Simpson HB, et al: Interpersonal functioning in obsessive-compulsive personality disorder. J Pers Assess 97(1):90–99, 2015 25046040

Chapman BP, Duberstein PR, Sörensen S, et al: Gender differences in five factor model personality traits in an elderly cohort: extension of robust and surprising findings to an older generation. Pers Individ Dif 43(6):1594–1603, 2007 18836509

Chavira DA, Grilo CM, Shea MT, et al: Ethnicity and four personality disorders. Compr Psychiatry 44(6):483–491, 2003 14610727

Chen C, Stevenson HW: Motivation and mathematics achievement: a comparative study of Asian-American, Caucasian-American, and East Asian high school students. Child Dev 66(4):1214–1234, 1995 7671657

Chess S, Clark KB, Thomas A: The importance of cultural evaluation in psychiatric diagnosis and treatment. Psychiatr Q 27(1):102–114, 1953 13014204

Church AT: Personality traits across cultures. Curr Opin Psychol 8:22–30, 2016 29506798

Costa PT, Terracciano A, McCrae RR: Gender differences in personality traits across cultures: robust and surprising findings. J Pers Soc Psychol 81(2):322–331, 2001 11519935

Eaton NR, Greene AL: Personality disorders: community prevalence and sociodemographic correlates. Curr Opin Psychol 21:28–32, 2018 28961462

Feingold A: Gender differences in personality: a meta-analysis. Psychol Bull 116(3):429–456, 1994 7809307

Fontenelle LF, Mendlowicz MV, Marques C, et al: Trans-cultural aspects of obsessive-compulsive disorder: a description of a Brazilian sample and a systematic review of international clinical studies. J Psychiatr Res 38(4):403–411, 2004 15203292

Grant BF, Hasin DS, Stinson FS, et al: Prevalence, correlates, and disability of personality disorders in the United States: results from the National Epidemiologic Survey on Alcohol and Related Conditions. J Clin Psychiatry 65(7):948–958, 2004 15291684

Grant JE, Mooney ME, Kushner MG: Prevalence, correlates, and comorbidity of DSM-IV obsessive-compulsive personality disorder: results from the National Epidemiologic Survey on Alcohol and Related Conditions. J Psychiatr Res 46(4):469–475, 2012 22257387

Hartung CM, Lefler EK: Sex and gender in psychopathology: DSM-5 and beyond. Psychol Bull 145(4):390–409, 2019 30640497

Kachel S, Steffens MC, Niedlich C: Traditional masculinity and femininity: validation of a new scale assessing gender roles. Front Psychol 7:956, 2016 27458394

Kanehisa M, Kawashima C, Nakanishi M, et al: Gender differences in automatic thoughts and cortisol and alpha-amylase responses to acute psychosocial stress in patients with obsessive-compulsive personality disorder. J Affect Disord 217:1–7, 2017 28363118

Kim J, Rapee RM, Ja Oh K, et al: Retrospective report of social withdrawal during adolescence and current maladjustment in young adulthood: cross-cultural comparisons between Australian and South Korean students. J Adolesc 31(5):543–563, 2008 18076980

McCrae RR, Terracciano A; Personality Profiles of Cultures Project: Universal features of personality traits from the observer's perspective: data from 50 cultures. J Pers Soc Psychol 88(3):547–561, 2005 15740445

McGilloway A, Hall RE, Lee T, et al: A systematic review of personality disorder, race and ethnicity: prevalence, aetiology and treatment. BMC Psychiatry 10:33, 2010 20459788

Mulder RT: Cultural aspects of personality disorder, in The Oxford Handbook of Personality Disorders. Edited by Widiger TA. New York, Oxford University Press, 2012, pp 260–287

Nemiah JC, Appel KE: Foundations of Psychopathology. New York, Oxford University Press, 1961

Nestadt G, Di CZ, Riddle MA, et al: Obsessive-compulsive disorder: subclassification based on co-morbidity. Psychol Med 39(9):1491–1501, 2009 19046474

Oltmanns TF, Powers AD: Gender and personality disorders, in The Oxford Handbook of Personality Disorders. Edited by Widiger TA. New York, Oxford University Press, 2012, pp 206–218

Paris J: Personality disorders in sociocultural perspective. J Pers Disord 12(4):289–301, 1998 9891284

Pollak JM: Obsessive-compulsive personality: a review. Psychol Bull 86(2):225–241, 1979 382220

Reas DL, Rø Ø, Karterud S, et al: Eating disorders in a large clinical sample of men and women with personality disorders. Int J Eat Disord 46(8):801–809, 2013 23983043

Samuel DB, Widiger TA: Conscientiousness and obsessive-compulsive personality disorder. Pers Disord 2(3):161–174, 2011 22448765

Schmitt DP, Realo A, Voracek M, et al: Why can't a man be more like a woman? Sex differences in big five personality traits across 55 cultures. J Pers Soc Psychol 94(1):168–182, 2008 18179326

Schmitt DP, Long AE, McPhearson A, et al: Personality and gender differences in global perspective. Int J Psychol 52(Suppl 1):45–56, 2017 27000535

Schulte Holthausen B, Habel U: Sex differences in personality disorders. Curr Psychiatry Rep 20(12):107, 2018 30306417

Schutter DJLG, Meuwese R, Bos MGN, et al: Exploring the role of testosterone in the cerebellum link to neuroticism: from adolescence to early adulthood. Psychoneuroendocrinology 78:203–212, 2017 28214680

Sprock J, Crosby JP, Nielsen BA: Effects of sex and sex roles on the perceived maladaptiveness of DSM-IV personality disorder symptoms. J Pers Disord 15(1):41–59, 2001 11236814

Terracciano A, McCrae RR: Cross-cultural studies of personality traits and their relevance to psychiatry. Epidemiol Psichiatr Soc 15(3):176–184, 2006 17128620

Weisberg YJ, Deyoung CG, Hirsh JB: Gender differences in personality across the ten aspects of the big five. Front Psychol 2:178, 2011 21866227

West C, Zimmerman DH: Doing gender. Gend Soc 1(2):125–151, 1987

Williams MT, Jahn ME: Obsessive-compulsive disorder in African American children and adolescents: risks, resiliency, and barriers to treatment. Am J Orthopsychiatry 87(3):291–303, 2017 27243576

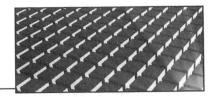

CHAPTER 8

PSYCHOBIOLOGY OF OCPD

Dan J. Stein, M.D.
Christine Lochner, M.D.

Case Vignette

Rodney is a 32-year-old man who was seen in our clinic after volunteering for research on siblings of individuals with obsessive-compulsive disorder (OCD). His younger brother had classic contamination obsessions and compulsive washing symptoms. Rodney denied ever having such symptoms but admitted that his living and work spaces were extremely orderly. Everything was in its place, and he preferred not to have people in his apartment and office because he would then have to rearrange everything after their departure. However, he indicated that his orderliness was useful for him and had no negative consequences because he simply met with people in other venues. On more detailed questioning, Rodney admitted that at times his pursuit of order and perfectionism interfered with his relationships: girlfriends had complained that he had difficulty showing warmth and that he was inflexible in his ways, and at work his supervisor complained that his approach to things slowed the team down. However, Rodney also felt that such accusations indicated a lack of insight, and he felt that he didn't need any psychological help. He indicated that he used a mental health app to do mindfulness meditation and that he followed its instructions to the letter, doing his meditation at the same time, and in the same way, every day.

Personality disorders, like other forms of psychopathology, can be conceptualized using categorical or dimensional approaches. Although these approaches are complementary (Kessler 2002), recent frameworks for neurobiological research have emphasized the value of dimensional investigations (Insel et al. 2010). In this chapter, we begin with a summary of neurobiological and neuropsychological work that has focused on obsessive-compulsive personality disorder (OCPD) as a diagnostic category. We then consider the neurobiology and neuropsychology of dimensions that may be particularly relevant to OCPD.

THE CATEGORY OF OCPD

Family Studies

Family studies have emphasized that relatives of individuals with a given psychiatric disorder may be more likely to suffer from subclinical symptoms or other *formes frustes* of the condition. From a neurobiological perspective, the genetic overlap in probands and relatives may lead to their sharing an intermediate phenotype, which may in turn increase risk for the illness (Gottesman and Gould 2003; Siever 2005). In a classic example from the personality literature, relatives of patients with schizophrenia are more likely to suffer from schizotypal personality disorder, and both conditions may be characterized by similar underlying neurobiological alterations (Grant et al. 2018).

Investigation of probands with obsessive-compulsive disorder (OCD) and their relatives has shown increased prevalence of OCPD in both probands and relatives as compared with healthy control subjects and their relatives (Samuels et al. 2000). Further, OCPD is more common in relatives of OCD probands than in relatives of control subjects (Bienvenu et al. 2012). There is also evidence from a number of studies that parents of children with OCD are more likely to have OCPD (Mancebo et al. 2005). Factor analysis of OCPD in families selected for having siblings with OCD found that OCPD symptoms comprise two factors: orderliness/perfectionism and hoarding/indecision (Riddle et al. 2016). A significant sibling-sibling correlation was found for the second factor but not the first, and this familial factor showed modest linkage to a region on chromosome 10 (Riddle et al. 2016).

Shared genetic and nonshared environmental factors contributing to OCD and OCPD were examined in a community sample of monozygotic and dizygotic adult twins (Taylor et al. 2011). The findings suggested that OC symptoms and traits were etiologically related primarily because they are shaped by the same nonspecific genetic factor that influenced negative emotionality. Although further nosological work is needed to disentangle the symptomatology of OCD and OCPD (Starcevic and Brakoulias 2017), family studies of OCD, including the one by Taylor et al. (2011), have been useful in understanding the neurobiology of OCPD, and we can be grateful to individuals such as Rodney for volunteering to participate in research.

What of OCPD in the general population? Twin studies have found that heritability of OCPD ranges from 27% to 78% (Reichborn-Kjennerud et al. 2007; Torgersen et al. 2000). Some work with twins has also found a single genetic factor that reflects a broad vulnerability to personality disorders and/or negative emotionality (Kendler et al. 2008). That said, data from these studies also showed that in terms of its underlying genetics, OCPD differs from other Cluster C disorders (Reichborn-Kjennerud et al. 2007) and has the highest disorder-specific loading (Kendler et al. 2008). Further work is needed, however, to determine whether there are differences in the neurobiology of OCPD in OCD probands and relatives versus OCPD in the general population.

Neuropsychological Studies

Several studies have examined whether neuropsychological dysfunctions characteristic of OCD are also seen in OCPD. On the basis of findings from their earlier work on patients with schizotypal and obsessive-compulsive personality traits (OCPTs), Aycicegi-Dinn and colleagues (2009) hypothesized that executive dysfunction would be demonstrated in individuals with OCPTs during neurocognitive task performance. The researchers administered the Rey-Osterrieth Complex Figure Test (ROCFT), a measure of executive control and working memory, to university students with OCPTs and healthy control subjects. Students with pronounced OCPTs had performance deficits, and such deficits were associated with OCPTs but not with OCD symptoms. The authors suggested that OCPTs may be a compensatory response to impaired executive control (Aycicegi-Dinn et al. 2009). García-Villamisar and colleagues found impairments on a range of tests of executive function in people with OCPTs. They argued that such dysfunction is consistent with clinical symptoms (García-Villamisar and Dattilo 2015) but also noted that such impairments are found in a range of personality disorders (Garcia-Villamisar et al. 2017).

Fineberg and colleagues administered tests of set shifting, executive planning, and decision making to individuals with OCPD and healthy control subjects (Fineberg et al. 2015). Individuals with OCPD had significant cognitive inflexibility as well as executive planning deficits but intact decision making. The authors emphasized that this neuropsychological profile is the same as that seen in patients with OCD and perhaps relatives of OCD probands and argued that this helps explain clinical symptoms of OCPD, including behavioral rigidity, perfectionism, and slowness (Fineberg et al. 2015). In an earlier study, Fineberg and colleagues also noted that patients with OCD and comorbid OCPD have even greater cognitive inflexibility than those without such comorbidity (Fineberg et al. 2007). The authors also found that individuals with OCPD may have relatively less difficulty with emotional processing than do those with OCD (Fineberg et al. 2015).

All of these studies were undertaken using community rather than clinical samples, which raises questions about the generalizability of findings. Paast et al. (2016) directly compared patients with OCD (and no OCPD), patients with OCPD, and healthy control subjects. They found that both patients with OCD and patients with OCPD had impaired cognitive flexibility and planning ability, with similar findings on most measures of these constructs.

Additional studies have explored a number of other cognitive-affective constructs. Pinto et al. (2014) found that compared with both patients with OCD and healthy control subjects, patients with OCPD had increased capacity to delay reward, which was associated with clinically significant perfectionism and rigidity. The authors argued that these findings are consistent with a view of OCPD as characterized by excessive self-control. Functional neuroimaging of delay discounting in healthy control subjects shows that selection of immediate rewards is associated with activation of limbic regions, including the ventral striatum and ventromedial cortex, whereas selection of larger delayed rewards is associated with activation of the dorsolateral prefrontal and parietal cortex. Given these findings, the authors suggested that future work imaging these brain areas in patients with OCPD during self-control tasks may be informative (Pinto et al. 2014). This conceptual framework certainly seems relevant to individuals such as Rodney. There is also an anecdotal literature on an association between OCPD and disgust (Pasquini et al. 2018), which deserves further elaboration, particularly given the putative role of disgust in OCD (Stein et al. 2001).

Neuroimaging and Molecular Studies

Although the literature on the use of neuroimaging in studies of personality disorders has expanded in recent years, there have been few neuroimaging studies of OCPD (Ma et al. 2016). A study of subjects with Cluster C personality disorders ($n=28$) found greater striatal surface area localized to the caudate tail, smaller ventral striatum volumes, and greater cortical thickness in right prefrontal cortex than in control subjects (Payer et al. 2015). A resting state functional magnetic resonance imaging (fMRI) study of a small group of individuals with OCPD found increased functional connectivity in the precuneus compared with healthy controls (Coutinho et al. 2016). The authors argued that, given that this posterior node of the default mode network is involved in self-reflection and in the retrieval of past events for current problem-solving and future planning, these findings are consistent with the characteristic rumination and perfectionism of OCPD.

A range of molecular systems play a role in neurocircuitry relevant to the neuropsychology and neuroimaging of OCPD, but to date there are few data on which to construct a neurobiology of OCPD. Findings of increased prevalence of OCPD in Parkinson's disease and supranuclear progressive palsy perhaps suggest a role for dopamine and striatal circuitry in OCPD, but it is also possible that such associations might involve other molecules and regions such as PTEN-induced kinase 1 (PINK1) and limbic circuitry (Nicoletti et al. 2015). Indeed, links between OCPD and various medical disorders do not necessarily lead to clear conclusions about relevant psychobiological mechanisms (Pasquini et al. 2014).

A study of salivary cortisol and α-amylase after the Trier Social Stress Test (TSST) in patients with OCPD suggested that males with OCPD responded with lower levels of these biomarkers than did healthy control subjects (Kanehisa et al. 2017). The authors suggested that these findings indicate attenuated sympathetic and parasympathetic activity in OCPD, but they also noted the limitations of this methodology. Data on response of OCPD to selective serotonin reuptake inhibitors (SSRIs) or other agents remain limited (Diedrich and Voderholzer 2015) and, in any event, point only indirectly to underlying molecular pathways.

Early genetic studies of OCD focused on specific candidate genes, including those in serotonergic and dopaminergic systems, but such studies have been criticized for statistical bias (Hemmings and Stein 2006). Indeed, candidate gene studies of serotonergic and dopaminergic gene variants do not provide very persuasive evidence of their role in OCPD without comorbidity (Joyce et al. 2003; Light et al. 2006; Perez et al. 2006). A postmortem study of gene expression in prefrontal cortex was undertaken in a group of patients including some with OCPD, but the number of OCPD individuals was low, and separate analyses of this group were not reported (Jaffe et al. 2014).

Genome wide-association studies (GWAS) provide an unbiased way of assessing genetic contributors to phenotypes. A GWAS of childhood OCPTs ($n=1,360$) found no significant hits, but three single nucleotide polymorphisms (SNPs) met the threshold of $P<10^{-5}$ (Boraska et al. 2012). A first SNP was in semaphorin 6D (*SEMA6D*); this gene belongs to the large semaphorin family and is involved in neural wiring of the central nervous system. A second was in Src homology 2 domain containing adaptor protein 4 (*SCH4*); this gene has previously been associated with depression. A third SNP lies close to disks large-associated protein 1 (*DLGAP1*); this gene plays an important role in glutamatergic function. Further work in larger samples is needed to replicate and extend these preliminary findings.

An early study compared serotonergic function, as assessed by prolactin response to fenfluramine, in males with OCPD, males with noncompulsive personality disorders, and healthy control subjects (Stein et al. 1996). Patients with OCPD had significantly blunted prolactin responses compared with noncompulsive patients and healthy control subjects. In the combined patient group, the total number of OCPTs correlated positively with impulsive aggression scores and inversely with prolactin responses. The authors argued that the data supported the hypothesis that impulsive and compulsive symptoms do not simply lie at opposite ends of a phenomenological and neurobiological spectrum but rather have a complex intersection, and both symptom types may correlate with serotonergic dysfunction (Stein et al. 1996). More recent neuroimaging and neurochemical studies provide some support for this hypothesis. These studies show that impulsive or compulsive behaviors are mediated by overlapping as well as distinct neural substrates, with serotonin and dopamine interacting across these circuits to modulate aspects of impulsivity and compulsivity (Fineberg et al. 2010, 2014). These findings provide an appropriate link to the next section on dimensions of OCPD.

DIMENSIONS OF OCPD

Work on the neurobiology of personality disorders has long suggested that different dimensions of personality can be distinguished on the basis of their underlying psychobiology (Siever and Davis 1991). Early work in this area suggested that anxious or inhibited individuals have specific physiological abnormalities, including increased tonic cortical arousal and sympathetic arousal, but decreased sedation thresholds and habituation to novel stimuli (Siever and Davis 1991). More recent work has focused on the neurobiology of personality dimensions such as neuroticism and harm avoidance.

The big five (or five-factor) model of personality has given impetus to a great deal of work on the dimensions of neuroticism, extroversion, openness to experience, agreeableness, and conscientiousness. Although there are some inconsistencies in the literature (Costa et al. 2005), OCPD may be characterized by increased neuroticism but also by increased conscientiousness and decreased agreeableness (De Fruyt et al. 2006). Furthermore, a twin study indicated a modest genetic correlation between OCD symptom dimensions and neuroticism (Bergin et al. 2014). Cloninger's model of personality traits has been particularly widely used in neurobiological research. OCPD may be characterized by increased persistence, as well as by decreased novelty seeking and reward dependence (De Fruyt et al. 2006). Also, parents of patients with OCD may have increased OCPD as well as increased harm avoidance (Calvo et al. 2009).

A number of imaging studies have focused on brain structures in neuroticism and harm avoidance (Servaas et al. 2013). A comprehensive literature review of this work found that neuroticism may be associated with individual differences in neurocircuitry involved in perception of and cognitive control over negative stimuli (Ormel et al. 2013). In particular, reduced connectivity between left amygdala and anterior cingulate cortex may be associated with impaired extinction of the amygdala response to anxiety-eliciting stimuli. Ormel et al. (2013) argued that these brain imaging findings are consistent with neuropsychological data indicating that neuroticism is associated with a negative bias in attention and in interpretation and recall of information and with increased reactivity and ineffective coping. Investigation of frontoamygdala activity in harm avoidance is ongoing (Baeken et al. 2014a; Kyeong et al. 2014).

Additional brain regions may also play a role in neuroticism and harm avoidance. In an fMRI study of a risk-taking decision-making task, right insula activation was stronger when subjects selected a "risky" rather than a "safe" response, and the extent of insula activation was associated with both neuroticism and harm avoidance scores (Paulus et al. 2003). The authors argued that insula activation serves as an aversive somatic markers, which in turn guides risk-taking decision-making behavior. An fMRI study of active versus passive avoidance found greater activation of the nucleus accumbens during active avoidance, with greater deactivation in passive avoidance (Levita et al. 2012). The authors concluded that the nucleus accumbens plays an important role in either emitting or withholding a response to avoid harm.

Neuroticism and/or harm avoidance have also been associated with brain alterations in a range of other areas, including dorsolateral prefrontal cortex, basal ganglia, and cerebellum (Forbes et al. 2014; Laricchiuta et al. 2014; Petrosini et al. 2017). It should also be noted that not all data are consistent. Liu and colleagues (2013) cautioned that the literature on the neuroanatomy of personality traits suffers from small sample sizes and from failure to control sufficiently for age- and sex-related effects. Collaborative networks that allow meta-analysis and mega-analysis of large data sets may be useful in addressing such criticisms (Thompson et al. 2015).

A range of molecular mechanisms in these various neurocircuits may contribute to neuroticism or harm avoidance. Molecular imaging investigations, for example, found that harm avoidance had negative correlations with dopamine $D_{2/3}$ receptor availability in striatal regions (Kim et al. 2011) and with serotonin transporter availability in midbrain (Wu et al. 2010) but positive correlations with serotonin type 2A (5-HT$_{2A}$) receptor binding indices in prefrontal regions (Baeken et al. 2014b) and with μ opioid receptor availability in a range of areas (Tuominen et al. 2012). However, these studies are limited by relatively small sample sizes. Reports that SSRIs or other medications improve neuroticism or harm avoidance are interesting, but again, they point only indirectly to the underlying psychobiology (Diedrich and Voderholzer 2015).

Meta-analyses of heritability of personality traits such as neuroticism and harm avoidance indicate moderate heritability across species, giving impetus to genetics research on these traits (Dochtermann et al. 2015; Sallis et al. 2018). A range of candidate gene studies have focused on dopaminergic and serotonergic genes in harm avoidance, but analyses are likely biased, and findings have been inconsistent (Balestri et al. 2014). Other genes that have preliminarily been associated with neuroticism or harm avoidance include brain-derived neurotrophic factor (Kim et al. 2010; Montag et al. 2010), neuropeptide Y (Zhou et al. 2008), GABA synthesis related enzyme GAD2 (Colic et al. 2018), cytokines such as γ-interferon (MacMurray et al. 2014), the estrogen receptor (Gade-Andavolu et al. 2009), cytochrome P450 2D6 (Roberts et al. 2004), neuroregulin 1 (Dina et al. 2005), and the MAM domain containing glycosylphosphatidylinositol anchor 2 gene (MDGA2 or MAMDC1) (Heck et al. 2011).

More recently a number of GWAS studies of neuroticism or harm avoidance have been undertaken (Sallis et al. 2018). In the largest of these studies to date ($n = 449,484$), a GWAS of neuroticism found 136 genome-wide significant loci. Analysis indicated enrichment involvement of specific cell types, including dopaminergic neuroblasts ($P = 3.49 \times 10^{-8}$), medium spiny neurons ($P = 4.23 \times 10^{-8}$), and serotonergic neurons ($P = 1.37 \times 10^{-7}$) (Nagel et al. 2018). Notably, polygenic risk score for neuroticism is associated with decreased cortical surface area in brain regions (i.e., precuneus and inferior parietal cortex) thought to be involved in internally focused cognition (Opel et al. 2018). However, in a smaller GWAS of Cloninger's personality dimensions, including harm avoidance and persistence ($n > 11,000$), no significant hits were found (Service et al. 2012).

Neuroticism and harm avoidance are the best studied personality dimensions that may be relevant to OCPD. Nevertheless, we note that there are also growing numbers of neuroimaging and neurogenetic studies of a range of other relevant phenotypes, including conscientiousness, perfectionism, self-control, and hoarding. See Chapter 12, "Positive Aspects of OCPD," for further discussion of conscientiousness. It is interesting, for example, that in a GWAS of conscientiousness, katanin catalytic subunit A1 like 2 (*KATNAL2*) reached significance; this gene is thought to play a role in cellular microtubule organization and has been linked with autism (de Moor et al. 2012). These investigations are potentially important for studying OCPD, and in the future it would be useful to link such work more directly to personality disorders.

PROXIMAL VERSUS DISTAL MECHANISMS

Biological explanations ought to explain not only the proximal mechanisms relevant to a particular phenotype (e.g., molecular mechanisms underlying personality traits) but also the distal mechanisms that have contributed to the ongoing persistence of relevant traits (e.g., evolutionary mechanisms relevant to personality traits). A number of evolutionary theorists have argued that different personality traits across species may be useful under different environmental conditions, with the consequence that a range of variation in personality persists in the population (Buss 1984, 2009; Dingemanse and Wolf 2010; Nettle 2006; Nettle and Penke 2010; Segal and MacDonald 1998).

An important framework in evolutionary theory contrasts slow and fast life history strategies. A slow strategy is characterized by low reproduction rates and high parental investment in offspring, whereas a fast strategy is characterized by high reproduction rates and low parental investment in offspring (MacArthur and Wilson 1967). Across species, a range of other variables correlate with choice of life strategy; for example, a slow life strategy is associated with greater weight at birth, longer time to mature, and longer lifespan (Stearns 1976). Each strategy involves a trade-off, having both advantages and disadvantages.

The life history framework has also been applied to explain individual differences, including personality traits (Del Giudice 2014). Impulsive personality traits are consistent with a fast life strategy, with its attendant advantages and disadvantages (Brüne 2016). Compulsive personality traits, on the other hand, are arguably compatible with a slow life history strategy, with its pros and cons. Hertler (2016) has applied this framework to OCPD, highlighting conscientiousness as a key characteristic of this disorder, and arguing that conscientiousness is the most robust personality marker of a slow life history strategy. He also suggested that other features of OCPD (e.g., harm avoidance, delayed gratification, hoarding) are consistent with a slow strategy.

The application of the life history conceptual framework to personality traits requires empirical support from animal and human investigations. To date, such support remains fairly limited. Nevertheless, there is a growing literature, including work on behavioral genetics, that specifically examines hypotheses that emerge from this framework and that provides some rationale for accepting some of its components (Gangestad 1997; Niemela and Dingemanse 2018).

CONCLUSION

Both categorical and dimensional approaches to OCPD and OCPTs have contributed to delineating the psychobiology of this disorder. Ongoing studies of these different approaches to OCPD and attempts to incorporate both approaches in neurobiological research on OCPD, OCD, and other putative obsessive-compulsive and related disorders is needed. Family studies suggest that at least some forms of OCPD are related to OCD, and neuropsychological studies have demonstrated overlaps in neuropsychological dysfunction in OCD and OCPD. Although these studies provide important clues regarding the neurocircuitry of OCPD, a lack of work on the neuroimaging and molecular biology of OCPD hampers the development of detailed models of its neurobiology. A range of brain structures, including amygdala and insula, may be involved in mediating OCPD-related personality traits, and there has been progress in delineating the genetic architecture of some of these substrates. The hope is that such work will ultimately contribute to assessment and intervention, but this goal may require much additional effort over many years before people such as Rodney benefit. Finally, biological explanations need to address both the proximal and distal mechanisms underlying different phenotypes. Further work on evolutionary approaches to OCPD may be useful for a more comprehensive understanding of the psychobiology of this condition.

TAKE-HOME POINTS

- At least some forms of OCPD are related to OCD, and there are overlaps in neuropsychological dysfunction in patients with OCD and OCPD.

- Specific brain structures, including the amygdala and insula, and a range of genes may mediate OCPD-related personality traits.

- There has been a paucity of research on the psychobiology of OCPD, and much additional work is required to advance the field.

REFERENCES

Aycicegi-Dinn A, Dinn WM, Caldwell-Harris CL: Obsessive-compulsive personality traits: compensatory response to executive function deficit? Int J Neurosci 119(4):600–608, 2009 19229723

Baeken C, Bossuyt A, De Raedt R: Dorsal prefrontal cortical serotonin 2A receptor binding indices are differentially related to individual scores on harm avoidance. Psychiatry Res 221(2):162–168, 2014a 24412555

Baeken C, Marinazzo D, Van Schuerbeek P, et al: Left and right amygdala—mediofrontal cortical functional connectivity is differentially modulated by harm avoidance. PLoS One 9(4):e95740, 2014b 24760033

Balestri M, Calati R, Serretti A, et al: Genetic modulation of personality traits: a systematic review of the literature. Int Clin Psychopharmacol 29(1):1–15, 2014 24100617

Bergin J, Verhulst B, Aggen SH, et al: Obsessive compulsive symptom dimensions and neuroticism: an examination of shared genetic and environmental risk. Am J Med Genet B Neuropsychiatr Genet 165B(8):647–653, 2014 25231027

Bienvenu OJ, Samuels JF, Wuyek LA, et al: Is obsessive-compulsive disorder an anxiety disorder, and what, if any, are spectrum conditions? A family study perspective. Psychol Med 42(1):1–13, 2012 21733222

Boraska V, Davis OS, Cherkas LF, et al: Genome-wide association analysis of eating disorder-related symptoms, behaviors, and personality traits. Am J Med Genet B Neuropsychiatr Genet 159B(7):803–811, 2012 22911880

Brüne M: Borderline personality disorder: why "fast and furious?" Evol Med Public Health 2016(1):52–66, 2016 26929090

Buss DM: Evolutionary biology and personality psychology: toward a conception of human nature and individual differences. Am Psychol 39(10):1135–1147, 1984 6507985

Buss DM: How can evolutionary psychology successfully explain personality and individual differences? Perspect Psychol Sci 4(4):359–366, 2009 26158983

Calvo R, Lázaro L, Castro-Fornieles J, et al: Obsessive-compulsive personality disorder traits and personality dimensions in parents of children with obsessive-compulsive disorder. Eur Psychiatry 24(3):201–206, 2009 19118984

Colic L, Li M, Demenescu LR, et al: GAD65 promoter polymorphism rs2236418 modulates harm avoidance in women via inhibition/excitation balance in the rostral ACC. J Neurosci 38(22):5067–5077, 2018 29724796

Costa PSJ, Bagby M, Daffin L, et al: Obsessive-compulsive personality disorder: a review, in Personal Disorders. Edited by Maj MA, Akiskal HS, Mezzich JE, et al. New York, Wiley, 2005, pp 405–477

Coutinho J, Goncalves OF, Soares JM, et al: Alterations of the default mode network connectivity in obsessive-compulsive personality disorder: a pilot study. Psychiatry Res Neuroimaging 256:1–7, 2016 27591486

De Fruyt F, De Clercq BJ, van de Wiele L, et al: The validity of Cloninger's psychobiological model versus the five-factor model to predict DSM-IV personality disorders in a heterogeneous psychiatric sample: domain facet and residualized facet descriptions. J Pers 74(2):479–510, 2006 16529584 de Moor MH, Costa PT, Terracciano A, et al: Meta-analysis of genome-wide association studies for personality. Mol Psychiatry 17(3):337–349, 2012 21173776

Del Giudice M: An evolutionary life history framework for psychopathology. Psychol Inq 25:261–300, 2014

Diedrich A, Voderholzer U: Obsessive-compulsive personality disorder: a current review. Curr Psychiatry Rep 17(2):2, 2015 25617042

Dina C, Nemanov L, Gritsenko I, et al: Fine mapping of a region on chromosome 8p gives evidence for a QTL contributing to individual differences in an anxiety-related personality trait: TPQ harm avoidance. Am J Med Genet B Neuropsychiatr Genet 132B(1):104–108, 2005 15578609

Dingemanse NJ, Wolf M: Recent models for adaptive personality differences: a review. Philos Trans R Soc Lond B Biol Sci 365(1560):3947–3958, 2010 21078647

Dochtermann NA, Schwab T, Sih A: The contribution of additive genetic variation to personality variation: heritability of personality. Proc Biol Sci 282(1798):20142201, 2015 25392476

Fineberg NA, Sharma P, Sivakumaran T, et al: Does obsessive-compulsive personality disorder belong within the obsessive-compulsive spectrum? CNS Spectr 12(6):467–482, 2007 17545957

Fineberg NA, Potenza MN, Chamberlain SR, et al: Probing compulsive and impulsive behaviors, from animal models to endophenotypes: a narrative review. Neuropsychopharmacology 35(3):591–604, 2010 19940844

Fineberg NA, Chamberlain SR, Goudriaan AE, et al: New developments in human neurocognition: clinical, genetic, and brain imaging correlates of impulsivity and compulsivity. CNS Spectr 19(1):69–89, 2014 24512640

Fineberg NA, Day GA, de Koenigswarter N, et al: The neuropsychology of obsessive-compulsive personality disorder: a new analysis. CNS Spectr 20(5):490–499, 2015 25776273

Forbes CE, Poore JC, Krueger F, et al: The role of executive function and the dorsolateral prefrontal cortex in the expression of neuroticism and conscientiousness. Soc Neurosci 9(2):139–151, 2014 24405294

Gade-Andavolu R, MacMurray J, Comings DE, et al: Association between the estrogen receptor TA polymorphism and harm avoidance. Neurosci Lett 467(2):155–158, 2009 19822194

Gangestad SW: Evolutionary psychology and genetic variation: non-adaptive, fitness-related and adaptive. Ciba Found Symp 208:212–223, discussion 223–230, 1997 9386914

García-Villamisar D, Dattilo J: Executive functioning in people with obsessive-compulsive personality traits: evidence of modest impairment. J Pers Disord 29(3):418–430, 2015 23445476

Garcia-Villamisar D, Dattilo J, Garcia-Martinez M: Executive functioning in people with personality disorders. Curr Opin Psychiatry 30(1):36–44, 2017 27798484

Gottesman II, Gould TD: The endophenotype concept in psychiatry: etymology and strategic intentions. Am J Psychiatry 160(4):636–645, 2003 12668349

Grant P, Green MJ, Mason OJ: Models of schizotypy: the importance of conceptual clarity. Schizophr Bull 44(suppl 2):S556–S563, 2018 29474661

Heck A, Pfister H, Czamara D, et al: Evidence for associations between MDGA2 polymorphisms and harm avoidance: replication and extension of a genome-wide association finding. Psychiatr Genet 21(5):257–260, 2011 21399569

Hemmings S, Stein D: The current status of association studies in obsessive-compulsive disorder. Psychiatr Clin North Am 29(2):411–444, 2006 16650716

Hertler S: The biology of obsessive-compulsive personality disorder symptomatology: identifying an extremely K-selected life history variant. Evolutionary Psychological Science 2:1–15, 2016

Insel T, Cuthbert B, Garvey M, et al: Research domain criteria (RDoC): toward a new classification framework for research on mental disorders. Am J Psychiatry 167(7):748–751, 2010 20595427

Jaffe AE, Deep-Soboslay A, Tao R, et al: Genetic neuropathology of obsessive psychiatric syndromes. Transl Psychiatry 4:e432, 2014 25180571

Joyce PR, Rogers GR, Miller AL, et al: Polymorphisms of DRD4 and DRD3 and risk of avoidant and obsessive personality traits and disorders. Psychiatry Res 119(1–2):1–10, 2003 12860355

Kanehisa M, Kawashima C, Nakanishi M, et al: Gender differences in automatic thoughts and cortisol and alpha-amylase responses to acute psychosocial stress in patients with obsessive-compulsive personality disorder. J Affect Disord 217:1–7, 2017 28363118

Kendler KS, Aggen SH, Czajkowski N, et al: The structure of genetic and environmental risk factors for DSM-IV personality disorders: a multivariate twin study. Arch Gen Psychiatry 65(12):1438–1446, 2008 19047531

Kessler RC: The categorical versus dimensional assessment controversy in the sociology of mental illness. J Health Soc Behav 43(2):171–188, 2002 12096698

Kim SJ, Cho SJ, Jang HM, et al: Interaction between brain-derived neurotrophic factor Val66Met polymorphism and recent negative stressor in harm avoidance. Neuropsychobiology 61(1):19–26, 2010 19923862

Kim JH, Son YD, Kim HK, et al: Association of harm avoidance with dopamine D2/3 receptor availability in striatal subdivisions: a high resolution PET study. Biol Psychol 87(1):164–167, 2011 21354260

Kyeong S, Kim E, Park HJ, et al: Functional network organizations of two contrasting temperament groups in dimensions of novelty seeking and harm avoidance. Brain Res 1575:33–44, 2014 24881884

Laricchiuta D, Petrosini L, Piras F, et al: Linking novelty seeking and harm avoidance personality traits to basal ganglia: volumetry and mean diffusivity. Brain Struct Funct 219(3):793–803, 2014 23494736

Levita L, Hoskin R, Champi S: Avoidance of harm and anxiety: a role for the nucleus accumbens. Neuroimage 62(1):189–198, 2012 22569544

Light KJ, Joyce PR, Luty SE, et al: Preliminary evidence for an association between a dopamine D3 receptor gene variant and obsessive-compulsive personality disorder in patients with major depression. Am J Med Genet B Neuropsychiatr Genet 141B(4):409–413, 2006 16583407

Liu WY, Weber B, Reuter M, et al: The Big Five of Personality and structural imaging revisited: a VBM–DARTEL study. Neuroreport 24(7):375–380, 2013 23531766

Ma G, Fan H, Shen C, et al: Genetic and neuroimaging features of personality disorders: state of the art. Neurosci Bull 32(3):286–306, 2016 27037690

MacArthur RH, Wilson EO: The Theory of Island Biogeography. Princeton, NJ, Princeton University Press, 1967

MacMurray J, Comings DE, Napolioni V: The gene-immune-behavioral pathway: gamma-interferon (IFN-γ) simultaneously coordinates susceptibility to infectious disease and harm avoidance behaviors. Brain Behav Immun 35:169–175, 2014 24075848

Mancebo MC, Eisen JL, Grant JE, et al: Obsessive compulsive personality disorder and obsessive compulsive disorder: clinical characteristics, diagnostic difficulties, and treatment. Ann Clin Psychiatry 17(4):197–204, 2005 16402751

Montag C, Basten U, Stelzel C, et al: The BDNF Val66Met polymorphism and anxiety: support for animal knock-in studies from a genetic association study in humans. Psychiatry Res 179(1):86–90, 2010 20478625

Nagel M, Jansen PR, Stringer S, et al; 23andMe Research Team: Meta-analysis of genome-wide association studies for neuroticism in 449,484 individuals identifies novel genetic loci and pathways. Nat Genet 50(7):920–927, 2018 29942085

Nettle D: The evolution of personality variation in humans and other animals. Am Psychol 61(6):622–631, 2006 16953749

Nettle D, Penke L: Personality: bridging the literatures from human psychology and behavioural ecology. Philos Trans R Soc Lond B Biol Sci 365(1560):4043–4050, 2010 21078656

Nicoletti A, Luca A, Luca M, et al: Obsessive-compulsive personality disorder in drug-naïve Parkinson's disease patients. J Neurol 262(2):485–486, 2015 25522699

Niemela PT, Dingemanse NJ: Meta-analysis reveals weak associations between intrinsic state and personality. Proc Biol Sci 285(1873):20172823, 2018 29491175

Opel N, Amare AT, Redlich R, et al: Cortical surface area alterations shaped by genetic load for neuroticism. Mol Psychiatry September 5, 2018 [Epub ahead of print] 30185937

Ormel J, Bastiaansen A, Riese H, et al: The biological and psychological basis of neuroticism: current status and future directions. Neurosci Biobehav Rev 37(1):59–72, 2013 23068306

Paast N, Khosravi Z, Memari AH, et al: Comparison of cognitive flexibility and planning ability in patients with obsessive compulsive disorder, patients with obsessive compulsive personality disorder, and healthy controls. Shanghai Jingshen Yixue 28(1):28–34, 2016 27688641

Pasquini M, Celletti C, Berardelli I, et al: Unexpected association between joint hypermobility syndrome/Ehlers-Danlos syndrome hypermobility type and obsessive-compulsive personality disorder. Rheumatol Int 34(5):631–636, 2014 24272065

Pasquini M, Maraone A, Roselli V, et al: Psychic euosmia and obsessive compulsive personality disorder. World J Psychiatry 8(3):105–107, 2018 30254981

Paulus MP, Rogalsky C, Simmons A, et al: Increased activation in the right insula during risk-taking decision making is related to harm avoidance and neuroticism. Neuroimage 19(4):1439–1448, 2003 12948701

Payer DE, Park MT, Kish SJ, et al: Personality disorder symptomatology is associated with anomalies in striatal and prefrontal morphology. Front Hum Neurosci 9:472, 2015 26379535

Perez M, Brown JS, Vrshek-Schallhorn S, et al: Differentiation of obsessive-compulsive-, panic-, obsessive-compulsive personality-, and non-disordered individuals by variation in the promoter region of the serotonin transporter gene. J Anxiety Disord 20(6):794–806, 2006 16303282

Petrosini L, Cutuli D, Picerni E, et al: Viewing the personality traits through a cerebellar lens: a focus on the constructs of novelty seeking, harm avoidance, and alexithymia. Cerebellum 16(1):178–190, 2017 26739351

Pinto A, Steinglass JE, Greene AL, et al: Capacity to delay reward differentiates obsessive-compulsive disorder and obsessive-compulsive personality disorder. Biol Psychiatry 75(8):653–659, 2014 24199665

Reichborn-Kjennerud T, Czajkowski N, Neale MC, et al: Genetic and environmental influences on dimensional representations of DSM-IV cluster C personality disorders: a population-based multivariate twin study. Psychol Med 37(5):645–653, 2007 17134532

Riddle MA, Maher BS, Wang Y, et al: Obsessive-compulsive personality disorder: evidence for two dimensions. Depress Anxiety 33(2):128–135, 2016 26594839

Roberts RL, Luty SE, Mulder RT, et al: Association between cytochrome P450 2D6 genotype and harm avoidance. Am J Med Genet B Neuropsychiatr Genet 127B(1):90–93, 2004 15108188

Sallis H, Davey Smith G, Munafo MR: Genetics of biologically based psychological differences. Philos Trans R Soc Lond B Biol Sci 373(1744):20170162, 2018 29483347

Samuels J, Nestadt G, Bienvenu OJ, et al: Personality disorders and normal personality dimensions in obsessive-compulsive disorder. Br J Psychiatry 177:457–462, 2000 11060001

Segal NL, MacDonald KB: Behavioral genetics and evolutionary psychology: unified perspective on personality research. Hum Biol 70(2):159–184, 1998 9549234

Servaas MN, van der Velde J, Costafreda SG, et al: Neuroticism and the brain: a quantitative meta-analysis of neuroimaging studies investigating emotion processing. Neurosci Biobehav Rev 37(8):1518–1529, 2013 23685122

Service SK, Verweij KJ, Lahti J, et al: A genome-wide meta-analysis of association studies of Cloninger's Temperament Scales. Transl Psychiatry 2:e116, 2012 22832960

Siever LJ: Endophenotypes in the personality disorders. Dialogues Clin Neurosci 7(2):139–151, 2005 16262209

Siever LJ, Davis KL: A psychobiological perspective on the personality disorders. Am J Psychiatry 148(12):1647–1658, 1991 1957926

Starcevic V, Brakoulias V: Current understanding of the relationships between obsessive-compulsive disorder and personality disturbance. Curr Opin Psychiatry 30(1):50–55, 2017 27755142

Stearns SC: Life-history tactics: a review of the ideas. Q Rev Biol 51(1):3–47, 1976 778893

Stein DJ, Trestman RL, Mitropoulou V, et al: Impulsivity and serotonergic function in compulsive personality disorder. J Neuropsychiatry Clin Neurosci 8(4):393–398, 1996 9116474

Stein DJ, Liu Y, Shapira NA, et al: The psychobiology of obsessive-compulsive disorder: how important is the role of disgust? Curr Psychiatry Rep 3(4):281–287, 2001 11470034

Taylor S, Asmundson GJ, Jang KL: Etiology of obsessive-compulsive symptoms and obsessive-compulsive personality traits: common genes, mostly different environments. Depress Anxiety 28(10):863–869, 2011 21769999

Thompson PM, Andreassen OA, Arias-Vasquez A, et al: ENIGMA and the individual: predicting factors that affect the brain in 35 countries worldwide. Neuroimage 145(Pt B):389–408, 2015 26658930

Torgersen S, Lygren S, Oien PA, et al: A twin study of personality disorders. Compr Psychiatry 41(6):416–425, 2000 11086146

Tuominen L, Salo J, Hirvonen J, et al: Temperament trait harm avoidance associates with μ-opioid receptor availability in frontal cortex: a PET study using [(11)C]carfentanil. Neuroimage 61(3):670–676, 2012 22484309

Wu IT, Lee IH, Yeh TL, et al: The association between the harm avoidance subscale of the Tridimensional Personality Questionnaire and serotonin transporter availability in the brainstem of male volunteers. Psychiatry Res 181(3):241–244, 2010 20153151

Zhou Z, Zhu G, Hariri AR, et al: Genetic variation in human NPY expression affects stress response and emotion. Nature 452(7190):997–1001, 2008 18385673

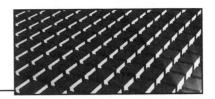

CHAPTER 9

PSYCHOTHERAPY FOR OCPD

Anthony Pinto, Ph.D.

Case Vignette

John, a 26-year-old graduate student, was asked to recount the various ways in which obsessive-compulsive personality disorder (OCPD) gets in the way of his life. Here is what he said (his original words have been edited for clarity):

"I guess as far back as I can remember, perhaps when I was 6 years old, I was preoccupied with order, how my room was organized, and how I had my toys set up. That's the way I liked it, and I would have a problem if my brothers or other people came into my room and placed things out of my order, the way I liked them. At that point, it was just with my things, and that didn't get in the way of my life. However, as I grew up and went to school, I definitely started to notice that I had a really big problem with procrastination on writing assignments. My high standards were getting in the way of completing assignments. So procrastination definitely started to show itself as I went through school.

"The most pervasive part of OCPD for me is the perfectionism and getting bogged down in the details of any assignment that I'm doing. If I feel like I am missing one minor detail, it gets in the way of completing the particular writing or research assignment. I really feel like I have to find that one thing before I can move on. With any paper I'm writing, I find myself stuck on page 1. I am often trying to get it just perfect before I can move on to the rest of the paper. I notice that with readings at school, it always takes me a lot longer to complete things than other people. I think I get obsessed with the details of the assignment or trying to understand every particular thing that I'm dealing with. One really good example is that I spend anywhere from a half hour to an hour writing an e-mail that would take most people 5 minutes to write. I make sure that all of my grammar and punctuation are perfect, that it says exactly what I wanted to say, and that it comes off just right. Especially in school, when working in groups, this has always been a huge problem for me. I never feel comfortable delegating anything to others and always think that my idea of how we should do the project is the way that it should be done. So naturally, there have been conflicts with that.

"Also, procrastination has been a huge problem for me. With every assignment, I say, "OK, this is not going to happen. I'm going to spend a lot of time on it, but I'm going to get this done in time." However, the very last day before the deadline arrives, and I'll be scrambling and doing it all at once. My goal is to try to make it great by spending a lot of time on it and doing it just the way I want. But instead, I end up pushing it off, and then it would be nowhere near what I want it to be.

"I have a lot of extremely high standards and I often hold my significant others to those high standards as well. I would be very argumentative with them. I would find anything that I thought we weren't seeing eye to eye on and really harp on that. If I noticed a flaw in them, I tended to focus on the flaws and ignore anything else that was good about them. Emotionally, it became very hard to express affection toward them. Even if I had negative emotions toward them, I was fearful of expressing those emotions as well.

"Even in my free time, when I'm doing something where I'm trying to enjoy myself, I feel like I have a really hard time being spontaneous. I feel like everything has to be planned out or I won't have a good time. I would be frustrated if a friend came up to me and said, "Hey, do you want to go grab drinks right now or go do something?" if it was something I hadn't planned on. If I didn't think things were set up to go right, I wouldn't have a good time.

"Doing any sort of chore is really a chore. It can be very frustrating, because with every little thing that I do, there's a right way to do it. If it's not done in that right way, then I get really upset. The best example might be the dishwasher. I always had this idea that the dishwasher had to be loaded in one particular way, and if it didn't get loaded in that way, then we were going to have horribly dirty dishes. I could not understand why any of my roommates didn't get that. So, anytime I would open the dishwasher, and they'd put something in there, I'd freak out and have to reorganize it. With shirts, I always had to have a perfectly ironed shirt before I could go into work. That's just the way it had to be. With a lot of things around my house, if I don't have control over it, it makes me very uneasy."

CORE FEATURES AND FUNCTIONAL IMPAIRMENT ASSOCIATED WITH OCPD

John describes several traits that are consistent with OCPD, a chronic condition that involves a maladaptive pattern of excessive perfectionism, preoccupation with orderliness and details, and the need for control over one's environment. In DSM-5 (American Psychiatric Association 2013), OCPD is defined as an enduring pattern that leads to clinically significant distress or functional impairment due to four or more of the following: preoccupation with details and order, self-limiting perfectionism, excessive devotion to work and productivity, inflexibility about morality and ethics, inability to discard worn-out or worthless items, reluctance to delegate tasks, miserliness toward self and others, and rigidity and stubbornness. Cognitive and behavioral features associated with OCPD include indecision (often related to the fear of making the wrong choice and often manifested through excessive research of decision options), difficulty coping with change in one's schedule or routine, being excessively rule-bound and wedded to routines, difficulty relating to and sharing emotions, anger outbursts when one's sense of control is threatened, and procrastination (usually linked to high standards of perfectionism). Through my clinical work, I have also noticed other particular features in patients with OCPD, such as a tendency to overexplain or overqualify statements with excessive details, a tendency to approach everyday tasks with such methodical intensity that progress is slowed or avoided and even leisure activities can feel like work, and a detail-oriented way of processing information that can slow down reading or lead to rereading passages or rewatching videos for fear of missing something.

DSM-5 reports that OCPD is one of the most common personality disorders in the general population, with an estimated prevalence ranging from 2.1% to 7.9% (American Psychiatric Association 2013). Individuals with this condition present frequently for treatment in both mental health (Bender et al. 2001) and primary care (Sansone et al. 2003) settings. However, OCPD remains an understudied phenomenon, and there is no definitive empirically supported treatment for this disorder.

OCPD traits are associated with significant functional impairment. The pursuit of perfection ends up being problematic (e.g., spending inordinate amounts of time on relatively trivial tasks, missing deadlines to write and rewrite assignments). Individuals with OCPD are typically seen as overly rigid and controlling because they often expect their coworkers, friends, and family to conform to their "right" way of doing things. They may also be inflexible about matters of morality and ethics and may attempt to impose their views on others. Consequently, individuals with OCPD often suffer from impaired interpersonal functioning, as well as high levels of internal distress (Cain et al. 2015). A study using well-validated measures of quality of life and psychosocial functioning found levels of impairment that were equivalent to levels in patients with obsessive-compulsive disorder (OCD; Pinto et al. 2014). In addition, a study of treatment-seeking patients with personality disorders found OCPD, along with borderline personality disorder, to be associated with the highest economic burden of all personality disorders in direct medical costs and loss of productivity (Soeteman et al. 2008).

As is true of other personality disorders, impaired interpersonal functioning is a hallmark feature of OCPD. Clinical descriptions indicate that interpersonal conflicts frequently occur among individuals with OCPD, often triggered by their impossibly high standards for the behavior of others, difficulty acknowledging differing viewpoints, and rigidity (Pollak 1987). Millon (1981) also noted that individuals with OCPD may be uncompromising and demanding, and OCPD has been linked with outbursts of anger and hostility, both at home and at work (Villemarette-Pittman et al. 2004). In a study investigating interpersonal functioning in OCPD, Cain et al. (2015) found that individuals with OCPD reported hostile-dominant interpersonal problems and a tendency to be overly controlling and cold in their relationships. OCPD was also associated with having a less empathic perspective relative to that of healthy control subjects, which may underlie some of the interpersonal problems described above. Cain et al. (2015) noted that individuals with OCPD "might have the capacity to experience sympathy and concern for others and might be able to intuit the appropriate affective response to another person…but are limited in their ability to subsequently demonstrate the appropriate emotional response in a social situation or adopt the other person's point of view" (p. 96).

Of the core features of OCPD, perfectionism has been highlighted in research and clinical reports as a major contributing factor to life impairment. *Maladaptive perfectionism*—the belief that anything less than perfect performance is unacceptable—has been linked to the development of depression (Rice and Aldea 2006). *Socially prescribed perfectionism*—the belief that one will be judged against unrealistic standards by others—has been linked to poorer relationship adjustment (Haring et al. 2003) as well as suicidal ideation (Hewitt et al. 1997). In fact, a diagnosis of OCPD may be a risk factor for suicidality, as declared by Diaconu and Turecki (2009), who found that among depressed patients, individuals with OCPD reported increased current and lifetime suicidal ideation, as well as a greater number of lifetime suicide attempts. Of special clinical concern, depressed patients with OCPD scored lower on the Reasons for Living Inventory and the Death Anxiety Questionnaire, both prognostic indicators of suicide.

Given that individuals can meet criteria for the disorder with any combination of four of the eight criteria, there is substantial heterogeneity within the OCPD population. On the basis of my clinical observations, there appear to be distinct OCPD subgroups. I have identified at least two such subgroups and refer to them as the hostile-dominant type and the anxious type. As presented in Table 9–1, these subgroups differ in their behavioral, cognitive, affective, and interpersonal profiles. For example, in the cognitive domain, hostile-dominant types are more likely to be mistrustful, to apply their high perfectionistic standards to both themselves and others, and to be somewhat eccentric, whereas anxious types are more likely to be self-critical, to apply perfectionistic standards to themselves, and to overattend to not meeting the expectations of others. Given the differences in presentation and potential functional impairment between these subgroups, the emphasis of psychotherapy in each case would also differ.

REVIEW OF PSYCHOTHERAPY RESEARCH FOR OCPD

Although there is no empirically validated gold standard treatment for OCPD, psychotherapy is recommended as the treatment of choice (Sperry 2003). The following subsections provide a review of the limited treatment research in OCPD.

Psychodynamic Psychotherapy

Psychodynamic treatment for OCPD involves an insight-oriented approach that attempts to reveal how the OCPD symptoms function to defend the individual against internal feelings of insecurity and uncertainty. When patients gain this insight, they then work to change their inflexible patterns of behavior and give up their rigid demands for perfection in favor of a more reasonable outlook. One study suggested that supportive-expressive psychodynamic therapy is effective for treating patients with OCPD and avoidant personality disorder (Barber et al. 1997). This study included 14 patients with OCPD and found significant improvement after 52 sessions but did not include a control group. In two subsequent trials of mixed personality disorder (including some individuals with OCPD), patients treated with brief psychodynamic treatments improved in terms of general functioning relative to waitlist control groups (Abbass et al. 2008; Winston et al. 1994); however, neither of these two studies specifically investigated improvement among those with OCPD, and the study outcomes did not assess for changes in OCPD symptoms specifically. Further research is needed to determine the effectiveness of psychodynamic treatments for OCPD.

TABLE 9–1.   Subgroups within OCPD

Profile	Hostile-dominant type	Anxious type
Behavioral	Workaholic	Workaholic
	Risk for self-harm	Procrastination
	Verbally hostile	Socially avoidant
		Sleep disturbance
Cognitive	Perfectionistic toward self and others	Perfectionistic toward self Self-critical
	Mistrustful Somewhat eccentric	Overattention to not meeting expectations of others
Affective	Irritable	Anxious
	Chronically frustrated Negative temperament	Somatic symptoms (e.g., irritable bowel syndrome)
	Difficulty with emotion regulation strategies and acceptance of emotion	Prone to worry, low mood
Interpersonal	Hostile, critical/judgmental	Submissive
	Rigid, controlling	Avoidance of intimacy
	Low empathy	
	Detached, emotionally unavailable	

Cognitive-Behavioral Therapy

Cognitive-behavioral therapy (CBT) typically involves a combination of both cognitive and behavioral techniques. The general cognitive therapy approach to treating OCPD involves identifying and restructuring the dysfunctional thoughts underlying maladaptive behaviors (Bailey 1998; Beck 1997; Beck and Freeman 1990). For example, patients would be taught to challenge "all-or-nothing" thinking by considering the range of possibilities that might be acceptable. Similarly, therapists might teach patients to recognize instances in which they overestimate the consequences of mistakes (catastrophizing) by examining the realistic significance of minor errors. CBT also includes behavioral elements, such as exposure to feared situations and stimuli through behavioral experiments (e.g., purposefully making small mistakes and observing the actual consequences) (Sperry 2003). Therapists may have difficulty establishing rapport with some OCPD patients because of their rigid thinking styles and difficulty with emotional expression. In light of this difficulty, Young's (1999) schema-focused therapy aims to identify and restructure patients' mal-adaptive schemas as they are expressed in the therapy process.

Although several cognitive and behavioral approaches to OCPD have been described (Kyrios 1998), very little empirical research has been conducted to test these treatments. In an uncontrolled trial conducted in patients from Hong Kong, Ng (2005) recruited individuals with treatment-refractory depression who also met DSM-IV criteria for OCPD (American Psychiatric Association 1994) and offered cognitive therapy focusing on the OCPD. Ten patients were treated, and after a mean of 22.4 sessions, all showed reductions in depression and anxiety symptoms, and nine no longer met diagnostic criteria for OCPD. However, this study did not include a control group and had a small sample size.

Strauss et al. (2006) conducted an open trial of cognitive therapy among outpatients with avoidant personality disorder ($n=24$) and OCPD ($n=16$) who received up to 52 weekly sessions. Results indicated that 83% of the patients with OCPD had clinically significant reductions in OCPD symptom severity and 53% had clinically significant improvement in depression severity. However, this open trial did not include a comparison condition, such as a waitlist control group or alternative treatment, precluding a firm conclusion about the efficacy of cognitive therapy for OCPD.

In the largest-ever trial of CBT for OCPD, Enero et al. (2013) enrolled 116 outpatients who met DSM-IV criteria for OCPD in an open trial of 10 weeks of group therapy for OCPD, consisting of psychoeducation, cognitive restructuring, behavioral experiments, and relapse prevention planning. The authors reported significant reductions in OCPD severity following treatment and found that pretreatment distress predicted OCPD response rate such that patients with lower levels of trait anxiety and depression were more likely to show a reduction in OCPD symptoms following treatment. However, a notable limitation of this trial is that it did not include a control group.

Very few studies have directly compared psychodynamic therapy and CBT to determine which is superior in the treatment of OCPD. In one study, Svartberg et al. (2004) randomly assigned patients with Cluster C personality disorders to receive 40 treatment sessions of either cognitive therapy ($n=25$) or short-term psychodynamic therapy ($n=25$). Avoidant personality disorder was the most frequent diagnosis in the sample, although OCPD was also represented, with eight individuals in the cognitive therapy group (32%) and nine in the psychodynamic group (36%) meeting DSM-III criteria for OCPD (American Psychiatric Association 1980. The results revealed that both treatment groups showed significant improvements on measures of symptom distress, interpersonal problems, and core personality pathology after treatment and at 2-year follow-up. There was no significant difference in improvement between the CBT and psychodynamic therapy groups across the full sample; however, the authors did not specifically compare treatment effects for the OCPD patients in particular. Thus, it is unclear whether CBT and psychodynamic therapy are equally effective, and more work is needed in this area.

Alternative Psychotherapies

Other treatments for OCPD have been explored in single-case studies. For example, two case studies have reported on adapting metacognitive therapy for individuals with OCPD (Dimaggio et al. 2011; Fiore et al. 2008). Metacognitive therapy aims to improve individuals' ability to understand mental states, enhancing awareness of their own emotions while also improving empathy and interpersonal functioning. This form of psychotherapy would seem well suited to the interpersonal problems frequently observed in individuals with OCPD, but more testing is needed. In one article, Lynch and Cheavens (2008) describe an adaptation of dialectical behavior therapy (DBT), now called Radically Open Dialectical Behavior Therapy (RO-DBT), designed to target cognitive rigidity and emotional constriction, and report on its successful implementation with one individual with OCPD. More recently, Lynch (2018) has put out a treatment manual for RO-DBT that focuses on treating disorders of overcontrol, including anorexia nervosa and OCPD.

Third-wave cognitive-behavioral treatments, such as acceptance and commitment therapy (ACT), have shown promise for the treatment of personality disorders (Ost 2008). ACT targets experiential avoidance by encouraging patients to accept and endure negative inner experiences (e.g., emotions, thoughts, memories) through the use of metaphors, mindfulness training, and behavioral therapy techniques. Applied to OCPD, ACT might involve educating patients about the paradoxical consequences of emotional avoidance (i.e., that attempts to control or eliminate unpleasant emotional states often amplify emotions and drive problematic coping strategies). Treatment would instead encourage individuals with OCPD to accept and tolerate negative emotional experiences rather than reacting in a controlling way. For example, patients could work to mindfully tolerate distressing emotions caused by imperfection and sudden changes in plans without immediately attempting to control the environment or situation. However, to date there have been no trials of ACT for OCPD.

A NOVEL PSYCHOTHERAPEUTIC APPROACH: TREATMENT FOR JOHN

My clinical experience, observations, and review of the literature point to the need to design novel treatments that challenge maladaptive perfectionism and rigidity and promote skills in healthy emotion regulation strategies and interpersonal functioning. As a result, in the case study of John presented in this chapter, I piloted a novel therapeutic intervention that consists of two established CBT modules: CBT for clinical perfectionism and rigidity preceded by skills training in emotion regulation and relationship flexibility.

Skills Training in Affective and Interpersonal Regulation (STAIR; M. Cloitre, K. Heffernan, L. Cohen, and L. Alexander: "STAIR/MPE: A Phase-Based Treatment for the Multiply Traumatized," unpublished manual, 2001; Cloitre et al. 2002) is a manualized form of CBT with two goals. The first is to learn how to experience feelings without becoming overwhelmed, which involves becoming more aware of feelings and what triggers them and learning how to manage certain emotions that can, at times, interfere with or overshadow relationship goals. A second goal is to improve interpersonal skills and use these skills flexibly and effectively in relationships. STAIR is administered with the intention of improving participants' current emotional and interpersonal functioning, as well as preparing them to fully utilize the subsequent CBT intervention.

CBT for clinical perfectionism and rigidity (Egan et al. 2014) has been tested in a series of studies (e.g., Egan and Hine 2008; Riley et al. 2007; Shafran et al. 2010). This manualized cognitive-behavioral approach consists of four aims developed originally by Fairburn et al. (2003): 1) identifying perfectionism as a problem and understanding maintaining mechanisms, including rigidity, overworking or overtraining, behavioral avoidance, dichotomous thinking, and cognitive biases; 2) conducting behavioral experiments to learn more about the nature of perfectionism and alternative ways of living; 3) psychoeducation and cognitive restructuring (in combination with behavioral experiments) to modify personal standards, self-criticism, rigid rules, and cognitive biases (e.g., selective attention to perceived failures); and 4) broadening the individual's scheme for self-evaluation by examining existing methods of evaluating the self and then identifying and adopting alternative cognitions and behaviors.

CASE STUDY: PRESENTING PROBLEM AND BACKGROUND

John (introduced in the case vignette at the beginning of this chapter) is a 26-year-old white male, never married, who is currently in graduate school and working at an internship. He lives with two roommates and has been in a romantic relationship for the past 9 months. His presenting problem is his preoccupation with lists, order, and perfectionism, which results in interpersonal problems and compromises his productivity. John presented with a neat appearance; full range of affect; euthymic mood; normal rate, tone, and volume of speech; linear thought process; appropriate thought content; and denial of suicidal ideation. John is not currently receiving any psychiatric or psychological treatment. He reports no psychiatric hospitalizations and has never had psychotherapy. His only prior treatment was use of a psychostimulant for about 1 year starting at age 25 (he stopped the medication 2 months prior to this evaluation). The medication was prescribed by a psychiatrist after John described trouble with focusing and completing tasks. John denies any chronic medical conditions, and his only medical hospitalization was for a tonsillectomy as a child.

CASE CONCEPTUALIZATION AND ASSESSMENT

At the evaluation visit, psychiatric and personality disorder diagnoses were confirmed by the Structured Clinical Interview for DSM-IV Axis I Disorders—Patient Version (SCID-I/P; First et al. 1996) and the Structured Clinical Interview for DSM-IV Axis II Personality Disorders (SCID-II; First 1997), respectively. John did not meet criteria for any affective, anxiety, psychotic, substance-related, somatic, or eating disorders. There was no evidence of attentional problems. John met criteria for OCPD and avoidant personality disorder. Using DSM-5, John meets the clinical threshold for six of the OCPD criteria.

1. Preoccupation with details and order: John devotes inordinate amounts of time to methodically compiling to-do lists that are counterproductive; must organize his work or home office space so that it is "just so" (e.g., computer charger is correctly positioned, coffee mug is in the correct spot) before he can be productive; and constantly looks for the best or most efficient way to do things (to the point of inefficiency). At work he has been given feedback that he is excessively attentive to superfluous details and late to turn in writing assignments because he insists on spending the bulk of time researching the topic and leaving little time to do the writing itself.
2. Self-limiting perfectionism: John has very high standards for the quality of his work (including e-mails, writing, and reading assignments)—everything must be done the "perfect way." He spends excessive time revising when writing (he estimates that he spends three to six times longer than his graduate school peers completing

writing assignments) and excessive time rereading assignments (he estimates that he takes twice as long to complete reading assignments as his graduate school peers). This difficulty completing tasks has significantly compromised his productivity at school and work.

3. Inflexibility about morality and ethics: John follows rules to the letter of the law, is angered and frustrated by those who do not adhere to rules (e.g., is distressed when he sees litter; becomes upset when someone at work leaves the door to the file room open because it contains confidential data). His girlfriend is turned off by his judgmental points of view; others often tell him that the things that upset him are "not a big deal."

4. Inability to discard: John has difficulty discarding items (e.g., clothing, textbooks, magazines, receipts, school papers), which has resulted in clutter that interferes with his living space.

5. Reluctance to delegate: John has difficulty delegating work because of concerns and frustrations that other people will not do it the right way. At school he resists group projects because of his tendency to butt heads with group members over the quality of the joint product. At home, he takes on most of the chores (e.g., cleaning, loading the dishwasher, caring for the dog) because he knows his roommates would not do them the way he wants. He often redoes others' work, which results in confrontations.

6. Rigidity and stubbornness: John's need to be methodical makes him resistant to change. He finds comfort in routines (e.g., he usually eats the same foods every day). He often insists on being right, even in areas in which there is no right answer. He frequently argues with others about being right, especially in romantic relationships, which has contributed to the demise of most prior dating relationships. At school, he becomes angry and resentful toward classmates and professors who have differing opinions.

John completed questionnaires about his OCPD symptoms, psychosocial functioning, emotion regulation, and interpersonal functioning at the orientation visit (week 0), after phase I (week 7), after phase II (week 14), and 2 months after acute treatment (week 22) (see Table 9–2).

The following measures were used in John's assessment:

The Social Adjustment Scale—Self Report (SAS-SR; Weissman and Bothwell 1976), a reliable, valid, and widely used self-report, measures current functioning in six domains: work, social and leisure, extended family, primary relationship, parental role, and family unit. An Overall Adjustment scale provides a total score based on the six domains. Higher scores on the SAS-SR indicate poorer functioning.

The Inventory of Interpersonal Problems—Short Circumplex (IIP-SC; (Hopwood et al. 2008) is a self-report measure of interpersonal prob-

TABLE 9–2.   Self-report measures completed by John and change scores by time point

Assessment measure	Baseline (week 0)	After phase I (week 7)	After phase II (week 14)	Two-month follow-up (week 22)	RCI (weeks 0–14)	RCI (weeks 0–22)
SAS-SR	3.16	1.73	1.58	1.38	**-4.27**	**-4.81**
IIP-SC Total	3.03	2	1.56	0.91	-1.47	**-2.12**
DERS Total	123	91	67	68	**-2.90**	**-2.85**
POPS Total	264	221	144	136	**-6.05**	**-6.45**
Difficulty with change	47	39	22	24	**-4.75**	**-4.37**
Emotional overcontrol	36	34	20	19	-1.71	-1.81
Rigidity	76	60	46	39	**-4.22**	**-5.20**
Maladaptive perfectionism	71	57	34	32	**-4.99**	**-5.26**
Reluctance to delegate	45	38	21	19	**-6.23**	**-6.75**

Note.   The reliable change index (RCI) was used to measure the change in scores on study measurements from pretreatment to posttreatment. Changes were assessed from baseline to week 14 and from baseline to week 22 (2-month follow-up). The RCI, which controls for initial severity and measurement error, is computed on the basis of the following general formula: $RCI = (x_2 - x_1) / s_{diff}$, where x_1 represents pretreatment scores, x_2 represents posttreatment scores, and s_{diff} is the standard error of difference between the pretreatment and posttreatment scores. The s_{diff} describes the spread of the distribution of change scores that would be expected if no actual change had occurred. RCI scores are scaled similarly to Z-scores. Therefore, RCI scores (absolute value) greater than 1.96 (given in bold) represent actual clinical change and are not attributed to variations of imprecise measuring instruments.
Abbreviations: DERS=Difficulties in Emotion Regulation Scale; IIP-SC=Inventory of Interpersonal Problems—Short Circumplex; POPS=Pathological Obsessive-Compulsive Personality Scale; SAS-SR=Social Adjustment Scale—Self-Report.

lems, with the following subscales: domineering, vindictive, cold, introverted, submissive, exploitable, overly nurturing, and intrusive. The total score represents an index of interpersonal distress across all types of interpersonal problems, with higher scores indicating greater distress.

The Difficulties in Emotion Regulation Scale (DERS; Gratz and Roemer 2004) assesses emotion regulation via a total score and six subscales: nonacceptance of emotional responses, difficulties engaging in goal-directed behavior when experiencing negative emotions, difficulties remaining in control of behavior when experiencing negative emotions, lack of emotional awareness, limited access to emotion regulation strategies, and lack of emotional clarity. Higher scores indicate more difficulties with emotion regulation.

The Pathological Obsessive-Compulsive Personality Scale (POPS; Pinto et al. 2011) is a 49-item self-report measure of maladaptive obsessive-compulsive personality traits and severity. Each item is rated on a 6-point scale ranging from 1 (strongly disagree) to 6 (strongly agree). A bifactor structure has been identified for this scale, consisting of five specific trait factors (rigidity, emotional overcontrol, maladaptive perfectionism, reluctance to delegate, and difficulty with change) and an overall factor (based on the total score) that represents obsessive-compulsive personality pathology on a continuum of increasing severity and dysfunction. The POPS has demonstrated excellent internal consistency reliability, as well as convergent and discriminant validity (Pinto et al. 2011; Wheaton and Pinto 2017). Wheaton and Pinto (2017) reported that POPS scores differentiate individuals who self-identify as having OCPD traits from community controls. In both the OCPD trait group and the community sample, greater severity of OCPD traits on the POPS was significantly negatively correlated with quality of life. The scale and a description are included in the appendix at the end of the chapter.

Initial impressions of John are that he is an intelligent and conscientious yet highly self-critical man experiencing major impacts on his functioning (as assessed by the SAS-SR) and interpersonal relationships (assessed by the IIP-SC) because of the domains of OCPD (assessed by the POPS) as well as his difficulties modulating negative emotions (assessed by the DERS). In terms of the subgroups described earlier in this chapter (see Table 9–1), John's presentation fits with the anxious type (e.g., workaholic, socially avoidant, self-critical, difficulties with time management).

Shafran et al. (2002) define *clinical perfectionism* as "the overdependence of self-evaluation on the determined pursuit of personally demanding, self-imposed standards in at least one highly salient domain, despite adverse consequences" (p. 778). The cycle of clinical perfectionism is maintained by cognitive biases (e.g., all-or-nothing thinking) and

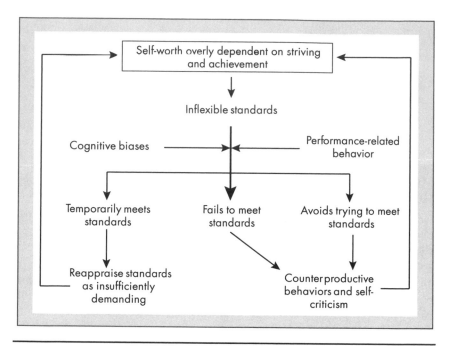

FIGURE 9–1.   The cognitive-behavioral model of clinical perfectionism.

Source.   From Shafran et al. 2010.

performance-related behaviors, including checking, being overly thorough, and avoidance or procrastination (see Figure 9–1 for illustration of this model and Figure 9–2 for its application to John). To bolster John's response to a targeted perfectionism intervention and strengthen his social supports, I decided to precede this intervention with a cognitive-behavioral skills building module (STAIR) that emphasizes increasing emotional awareness and instilling greater relationship flexibility.

TREATMENT COURSE

The 14-week treatment protocol for John consisted of 15 sessions: an orientation visit, STAIR (phase I, comprising six weekly sessions), and CBT for perfectionism and rigidity (phase II, with eight weekly sessions). The session-by-session protocol is described in the following subsections, including the agenda for each session and notes on John's progress in treatment.

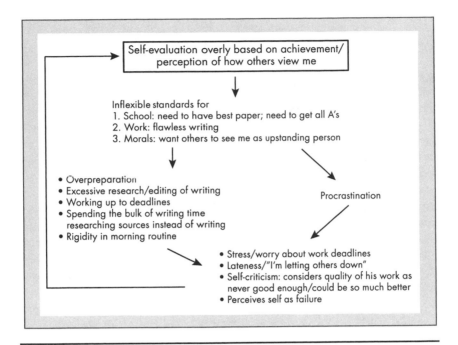

FIGURE 9–2. The cognitive-behavioral model of perfectionism, adapted for John.

Orientation Session

During the orientation session, I reviewed the treatment rationale and targets for phases I and II, as well as psychoeducation about OCPD and related functional impairment.

Phase I: STAIR Treatment (Weeks 1–6)

The first phase of the treatment consisted of six sessions of STAIR (each 50 minutes long). STAIR sessions have essentially the same format: 1) psychoeducation about relationships and interpersonal skills deficits, 2) identification of strengths and weaknesses related to a given skill, 3) illustration of the new skill, and 4) practice of the new skill. John was given a session outline handout at the end of each STAIR session so he could review the psychoeducation and skills training from each session at home. At the end of each session, I assigned John between-session work that consisted of exercises directly related to the content of the given session. At the beginning of each session, John and I reviewed between-session work from the previous week and addressed difficulties in implementing new coping skills. The six STAIR sessions followed a conceptual progression from a focus on basic identification and labeling of emotions to a review of the importance of emotions in interpersonal relationships to a focus on interpersonal flexibility.

Session 1: Introduction to Treatment Rationale

During session 1, John received psychoeducation about emotion regulation. In addition, John practiced self-monitoring of feelings and labeling of emotions. I introduced a self-monitoring form and demonstrated its use by asking John to identify a time in the past week when strong feelings were triggered. John rated the intensity of the feeling and identified the situation or trigger. The importance of self-monitoring throughout phase I of this treatment was emphasized, and I gave John a list of feelings words to aid in identifying his emotions. Breathing retraining (with emphasis on slow, rhythmic diaphragmatic breathing) was demonstrated and practiced.

Homework 1: Breathing retraining practice for 5 minutes twice daily; self-monitoring of feelings.

Session 2: Emotion Regulation

In session 2, we began by reviewing the self-monitoring form that John completed between sessions and checked on the breathing exercise he completed. Psychoeducation in this session covered negative mood regulation; the connection between feelings, thoughts, and behaviors; and a discussion of John's current coping skills. John also learned about identifying the three channels of distress: physiological, cognitive, and behavioral (Figure 9–3), as well as new coping skills for intervening at each channel.

Homework 2: Breathing retraining; self-monitoring; practice of new coping skills for cognitive channel (e.g., positive images and self-statements and shifting attention during stressful events).

Session 3: Distress Tolerance

During session 3, we reviewed the feelings self-monitoring form and alternative coping methods. Psychoeducation for this week explored acceptance of feelings and distress tolerance, and to illustrate this we completed an exercise on assessing pros and cons of an identified goal and coping with the associated distress (using a decisional balance form). John focused on the pros and cons of making contact with a former supervisor because he worried she might focus on a deadline he had missed during the time he had worked for her. John concluded that making the contact would be beneficial for his career, despite the distress and shame he would endure. He and I also identified pleasurable

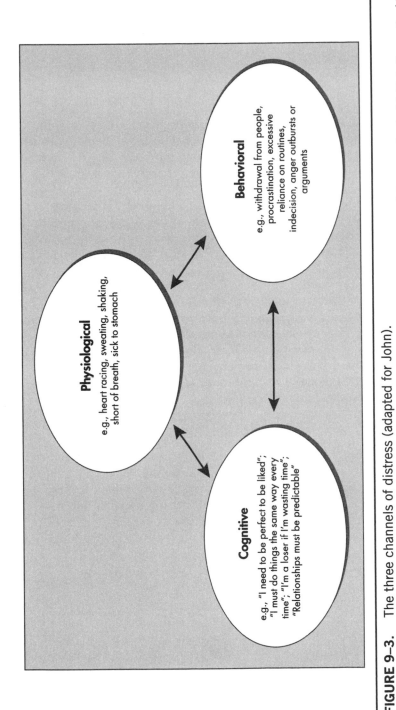

FIGURE 9–3. The three channels of distress (adapted for John).

Source. Adapted from M. Cloitre, K. Heffernan, L. Cohen, and L. Alexander: "STAIR/MPE: A Phase-Based Treatment for the Multiply Traumatized." Unpublished manual, 2001.

activities (from a list of suggestions), including riding his bicycle and making plans with friends.

Homework 3: Breathing retraining; self-monitoring; assessment of pros and cons of entering one difficult situation and tolerating distress; use of new skills to manage distress; engaging in pleasurable activities.

Session 4: Relationship Between Affect and Interpersonal Problems

In session 4, we reviewed the feelings self-monitoring form. John was reinforced for trying alternative means of coping with distress, and we discussed positive activities that he had explored in the past week. John noted that his former supervisor was very happy to hear from him and that she was highly complimentary of his work and expressed interest in working with him again. She made no mention of the missed deadline and may not have even been aware of it. Psychoeducation for session 4 focused on interpersonal schemas (organizing templates, expectations, and beliefs about relationships and how they work) and included an exercise on identifying interpersonal schemas by using an interpersonal schema worksheet. One of the primary goals of STAIR is helping individuals to identify the interpersonal schemas that are coming into play in current relationships and causing problems in their interpersonal functioning. John discussed his insistence on doing all aspects of a job himself (at his internship and at home) and how this view may affect how others perceive him.

Homework 4: Breathing retraining; self-monitoring; interpersonal schema worksheet once daily.

Session 5: Alternative Interpersonal Schemas

In session 5, John and I reviewed feelings monitoring and alternative coping, and I gave him feedback on his attempts to complete the interpersonal schema worksheet. Role-play was presented as a powerful therapy tool. We identified a relevant interpersonal situation (a perceived conflict with a peer in his graduate program) and conducted three consecutive iterations of the role-play: 1) John being himself and me playing the other person, 2) me playing John and John playing the other person, and 3) a switch back to John as himself and me as the other person. This approach allowed me to give John immediate feedback on his interpersonal skills and ways to make his communication more effective, which he was then able to practice. We discussed generating alternative schemas to interpersonal situations and applied the role plays to the interpersonal schema worksheet. John also learned how to use covert modeling (imagining oneself in an interaction) as another tool for coming up with alternative responses when role-play is not possible.

Homework 5: Breathing retraining; self-monitoring; initiating at least one interpersonal situation to practice using an alternative approach.

Session 6: Interpersonal Flexibility

During session 6, we reviewed feelings monitoring and alternative coping, as well as John's attempts to complete the interpersonal schema worksheet. This session's psychoeducation was about various types of power balances in relationships (equal power relationships, relationships in which one has more power than the other, and relationships in which one has less power than the other) and the importance of flexibility and adaptability in interpersonal situations. To demonstrate this, we conducted role-plays for different power balances in John's life. Last, we discussed the transition to phase II of treatment: CBT for perfectionism and rigidity.

Homework 6: Self-monitoring; interpersonal schema worksheet once daily; practice using interpersonal flexibility with different power differentials; list of questions and concerns regarding transition to phase II.

Phase II: CBT for Clinical Perfectionism and Rigidity (Weeks 7–14)

The second phase of John's treatment consisted of eight sessions of CBT for perfectionism and rigidity (each 50 minutes long). Throughout phase II, John was assigned to read sections from the book *Overcoming Perfectionism* (Shafran et al. 2010). Between-session work was assigned at the end of each session and consisted of exercises directly related to the content of the given session. Between-session work from the previous week was reviewed at the beginning of each session, and difficulties in implementing exercises were addressed.

Session 7: Cognitive-Behavioral Formulation and Psychoeducation

We began session 7 by reviewing the highlights of phase I. John noted that he benefited from learning to better verbalize his emotions, knowing how and when to apply assertiveness to interactions, identifying interpersonal goals, being flexible with regard to different power differentials in interactions, and challenging assumptions that arise from interpersonal schemas. Phase II of treatment was introduced. John and I reviewed the main domain(s) of John's psychosocial functioning impacted by perfectionism and discussed examples. We also reviewed the cognitive-behavioral model of perfectionism (see Figure 9–1) and how it is maintained from a case example, and then we drew the model on the basis of John's own life (see Figure 9–2). We also discussed the pros and cons of perfectionism and making changes, and I assigned readings for homework.

Session 8: Self-Monitoring and Myths Regarding Perfectionism

In session 8, we discussed John's questions about reading assignments and then reviewed key points about self-monitoring. We generated a list of behaviors that were contributing to John's clinical perfectionism (e.g., list making, checking or going over work mentally, avoidance and procrastination, not deviating from routines). John was assigned to monitor specified behaviors for homework. Next, John identified areas of his life that have been affected by his perfectionism, and we practiced self-monitoring of perfectionism-related thoughts, standards, emotions, and behaviors. Finally, we reviewed a list of myths relevant to perfectionism (e.g., "Successful people work harder than less successful people"; "To get ahead, you have to be single-minded and give up all outside interests"). In addition to self-monitoring and reading his assignment, John was asked to complete a questionnaire about the frequency of various perfectionism-related behaviors (e.g., "How often do you check your work for mistakes?").

Session 9: Surveys and Behavioral Experiments

In session 9, we reviewed the questionnaire and self-monitoring forms assigned in session 2 and then discussed the rationale for using surveys in John's treatment as a means of learning how others cope with some of the standards John has been struggling with. For example, writing research papers is a particular challenge for John. Because of his need to make sure he has done an exhaustive review of the academic literature, he would spend so much time researching the topic that little time would be left for the actual writing. We decided to create a survey that he would give to graduate school peers so that he could better understand how much time and effort his colleagues were putting into their research papers (e.g., how long they spent looking for articles and references vs. writing). We discussed the rationale for behavioral experiments and discussed a case example. We then set up a behavioral experiment for John's homework: going to work without ironing his shirt to see if anyone noticed. Setting up the experiment included specifying the belief or standard to be tested, the prediction, and the approach. John agreed to note the results and to reflect on how they relate to his prediction.

Session 10: Challenging Dichotomous Thinking via Behavioral Experiments

We began session 10 by reviewing the outcomes of the survey and behavioral experiment. John was fascinated to hear his graduate school peers' methods for doing research papers. He noted that learning the methods of his most respected peers gave him further insight about the inefficiency of his approach to writing papers. John also completed the behavioral experiment, and, contrary to his prediction, there were no reactions to his wrinkled shirt, and the outcome of his day did not appear to be affected by the shirt. After reviewing this experiment, I provided psychoeducation about dichotomous (all-or-nothing) thinking. To explore this further, we set up a behavioral experiment for all-or-nothing thinking: John agreed to test his belief that if he cannot outline all of the assigned chapters for a class, he might as well wait until the exam to do it. In this experiment, he agreed to outline one chapter. I also introduced continua to emphasize flexible thinking.

Session 11: Challenging Cognitive Biases

In session 10, we focused on cognitive biases such as selective attention to the negative, discounting positive aspects of performance, double standards and accompanying self-criticism, and overgeneralization. These cognitive maintenance factors of clinical perfectionism and rigidity were addressed using behavioral experiments in addition to cognitive restructuring (using thought diaries). John also reported on a self-initiated behavioral experiment: On 3 nights over the previous week, he made a point of going to sleep before his roommates to test whether they would lock up and turn off the lights (tasks he usually took on himself because of his concern that his roommates would not). He reported that, contrary to his prediction, his roommates did take on these tasks when he went to sleep. On reflection, John was relieved that he would no longer have to be the last to bed.

Session 12: Procrastination, Time Management, and Pleasant Events

We began session 12 with psychoeducation about procrastination, its relationship to perfectionism, and the benefits and costs associated with it. We then identified areas of procrastination in John's life, particularly with his school work, preparing for exams, and writing research papers. We discussed problem-solving approaches to procrastination, including the technique of breaking tasks into manageable chunks, and applied this to an upcoming group project for one of his classes. We discussed time management, activity scheduling, and balancing achievement and fun. We reviewed a possible time management schedule, blocking out study time versus leisure. John agreed to do a behavioral experiment to test his belief that activities that are not planned out are a waste of time: he agreed to ride his bike around the city without a planned destination.

Session 13: Self-Criticism and Self-Compassion

In session 13, John reported completing the behavioral experiment and enjoying his bike ride. He concluded that even spontaneous, unplanned activities can be worthwhile. I checked in regarding his group project and his attempt at breaking down the assignment into manageable chunks. We discussed the problem of self-criticism and how it stems from trying to adhere to rigid and demanding rules as well as extreme personal standards for performance. An overarching goal of this phase includes encouraging the patient to relax rules for performance (i.e., do things well enough), replace rules with guidelines (i.e., do things flexibly), and avoid generalizing poor performance on a task to negative judgments about self-worth. I presented a story about two coaches, one who is highly critical and hostile and another who is more compassionate. We discussed which coach in the analogy would coax better performance from athletes. Afterward, we practiced thought records for self-critical and compassionate thoughts, and I explained the concept of treating oneself as one would treat a friend. Related worksheets were assigned.

Session 14: Self-Evaluation and Relapse Prevention

In session 14, we reviewed John's final homework assignments and then discussed the final psychoeducation topic: self-evaluation and how to broaden it to various life areas rather than just achievement. We reflected on John's strong progress in treatment and changes that he wants to continue to develop in line with his goals and values. We also discussed relapse prevention and preparing for potential setbacks.

Over the 14 weeks of treatment, John showed clinically significant improvement and no longer met diagnostic criteria for OCPD at the end of phase II. His improvement was further demonstrated by the robust change in his scores, as indicated by significant reliable change indices, on the OCPD and functioning measures (see Table 9–2). This improvement was maintained at the 2-month follow-up assessment. At the follow-up appointment, I asked John to comment on his progress and what treatment components were helpful. Here is his response:

> The first thing that has been very helpful is with regulating my emotions. I guess it's funny, because until treatment began, I would often find that when asked how I'm feeling or what my emotions were like, I wouldn't know. I would just say, "I'm not sure what I'm feeling." I always had a hard time expressing them. But now, I think the treatment has greatly helped me to become more emotionally aware, and aware of what I'm feeling, and to be able to write out what I'm feeling at a particular time. It has been very helpful to connect the feelings I'm having with the thoughts I'm having—for example, why I am feeling a particular way, and why the thought that I'm having in my head is leading to that feeling. So, the emotional part has been very helpful.
>
> Also, it has been really helpful to test these high standards I have, and to do these experiments with myself. For example, if I think that

whatever I'm doing has to be done in a particular way, or has to meet a standard, I can test that, and discover that it's OK not to do it that way. It has been great. For instance, with my leisure time, I always thought that everything had to be specifically planned or I wasn't going to enjoy myself. But I did experiments where I went out without a plan, and I had a wonderful time enjoying myself. Another example is with ironing my shirts—I thought that if I went to work with a wrinkled shirt, everyone would think I was a fool, I'd be embarrassed, and it would just be horrible. However, I went to work with a wrinkled shirt one day, and the world didn't explode. Everything was great, I had a great day at work, and nobody seemed to notice. So those are the biggest things that have been really helpful in overcoming a lot of this. I'm really grateful for this opportunity. I've seen a huge improvement.

CONCLUSION

OCPD is marked by the core features of self-limiting perfectionism and rigidity. Individuals with OCPD report significant impairment in psychosocial functioning and quality of life. Despite the prevalence of OCPD in the general population and the high rates of treatment utilization by these patients, there is no definitive empirically supported treatment for the condition. In this chapter, I outline a novel pilot psychotherapy that addresses not only the core symptoms of OCPD but also problems with emotion regulation and interpersonal functioning. This 14-week treatment consists of two established manualized CBT components: 1) the skills building module (STAIR) that emphasizes increasing emotional awareness and instilling greater relationship flexibility and 2) CBT for perfectionism and rigidity, which targets the maintaining mechanisms in the clinical perfectionism model—namely, cognitive biases, counterproductive behaviors, rigid rules and standards, and punishing self-criticism.

OCPD remains an underrecognized phenomenon in the community. For example, a community survey found very low recognition rates for OCPD, with participants much more likely to correctly identify depression, schizophrenia, and OCD (Koutoufa and Furnham 2014). Clinicians should be aware of the core features and symptomatic behaviors of OCPD so that they can assess for them and address them in psychotherapy. In the case of John, his "trouble with focusing and completing tasks" had been previously mislabeled and treated as an attentional problem.

In the early stages of psychotherapy for OCPD, clinicians should assess the patient's level of self-care, including quality of eating, sleep, physical activity, and social activity and leisure. The patient's level of self-care may be adversely impacted because of his or her difficulty with time management and procrastination, overattention to work or productivity, and negative self-evaluation. By problem solving ways to bolster each of these self-care domains, the patient will lower his or her vulnerability to distress and low mood, as well as increase the mental resources available for making behavioral changes.

When treating a patient with OCPD, the clinician needs to convey that the objective of CBT targeting the clinical perfectionism model is not to remove the individual's standards for performance or to turn the individual into someone who settles for mediocrity. Instead, the objective is to relax the individual's rigid internalized rules (i.e., to aim for "good enough" instead of perfection) and replace them with guidelines that allow for greater flexibility and efficiency while triggering less harsh self-criticism.

Throughout the process of psychotherapy for OCPD, the clinician should engage the patient in identifying his or her values and considering how OCPD traits are interfering in the patient's ability to move in the direction of those values. To be effective, the clinician must convey how making behavioral changes in the context of the therapy will bring the patient closer to his or her values. For example, when working on time management or activity planning, the patient will be encouraged to allocate time in his or her schedule in a way that maps on to his or her values. When working on decision making, the patient will be encouraged to prioritize a particular value and practice making decisions in the service of that value.

John, a 26-year-old graduate student, presented for treatment because of major impacts on his functioning and interpersonal relationships from his intense perfectionism and rigidity as well as his difficulties modulating negative emotions. John was clearly motivated and open to change. He embraced the treatment and followed through on between-session practice. His response to treatment was clinically significant, as evidenced by his diagnostic remission at the conclusion of treatment as well as the robust improvement in scores on the OCPD and functioning measures, which was maintained at 2 months posttreatment. This is notable considering that OCPD has at times been dismissed as an unchangeable personality condition. Although this pilot offers a promising lead for further study, much more systematic research is needed to further develop treatments for this disorder.

TAKE-HOME POINTS

- Even in the absence of a categorical diagnosis of OCPD, clinically significant traits such as perfectionism and rigidity can interfere in the treatment of anxiety and mood conditions.

- In the early stages of psychotherapy for OCPD, clinicians should assess the patient's level of self-care, including quality of eating, sleeping, physical activity, and social activity or leisure.

- Skills training in modulating negative emotions and applying flexibility to relationships may be key components in treating OCPD because they may allow these individuals to better access support.

- The objective of psychotherapy for OCPD is to help the individual learn about his or her rigid internalized rules and replace them with guidelines that allow for greater flexibility and efficiency while triggering less harsh self-criticism.

- Behavioral experiments can be an effective way to test perfectionism standards because they allow the individual to objectively collect his or her own data (in the real world) as to the validity of the standard and the likelihood of the unwanted outcome.

- In order for treatment to be effective, the clinician must convey how making behavioral changes in the context of the therapy will bring the patient closer to his or her values.

REFERENCES

Abbass A, Sheldon A, Gyra J, et al: Intensive short-term dynamic psychotherapy for DSM-IV personality disorders: a randomized controlled trial. J Nerv Ment Dis 196(3):211–216, 2008 18340256

American Psychiatric Association: Diagnostic and Statistical Manual of Mental Disorders, 3rd Edition. Washington, DC, American Psychiatric Association, 1980

American Psychiatric Association: Diagnostic and Statistical Manual of Mental Disorders, 4th Edition. Washington, DC, American Psychiatric Association, 1994

American Psychiatric Association: Diagnostic and Statistical Manual of Mental Disorders, 5th Edition. Arlington, VA, American Psychiatric Association, 2013

Bailey GR Jr: Cognitive-behavioral treatment of obsessive-compulsive personality disorder. J Psychol Pract 4(1):51–59, 1998

Barber JP, Morse JQ, Krakauer I, et al: Change in obsessive-compulsive and avoidant personality disorders following time-limited supportive-expressive therapy. Psychotherapy 34:133–143, 1997

Beck AT, Freeman A: Cognitive Therapy of Personality Disorders. New York, Guilford, 1990

Beck JS: Cognitive approaches to personality disorders, in Cognitive Therapy. Edited by Wright JH, Thase ME. Review of Psychotherapy Series, Vol 16, No 1; Dickstein LJ, Riba MB, Oldham JO, series eds. Washington, DC, American Psychiatric Press, 1997, pp 73–106

Bender DS, Dolan RT, Skodol AE, et al: Treatment utilization by patients with personality disorders. Am J Psychiatry 158(2):295–302, 2001 11156814

Cain NM, Ansell EB, Simpson HB, et al: Interpersonal functioning in obsessive-compulsive personality disorder. J Pers Assess 97(1):90–99, 2015 25046040

Cloitre M, Koenen KC, Cohen LR, et al: Skills training in affective and interpersonal regulation followed by exposure: a phase-based treatment for PTSD related to childhood abuse. J Consult Clin Psychol 70(5):1067–1074, 2002 12362957

Diaconu G, Turecki G: Obsessive-compulsive personality disorder and suicidal behavior: evidence for a positive association in a sample of depressed patients. J Clin Psychiatry 70(11):1551–1556, 2009 19607764

Dimaggio G, Carcione A, Salvatore G, et al: Progressively promoting metacognition in a case of obsessive-compulsive personality disorder treated with metacognitive interpersonal therapy. Psychol Psychother 84(1):70–83, 98–110, 2011 22903832

Egan SJ, Hine P: Cognitive behavioural treatment of perfectionism: a single case experimental design series. Behaviour Change 25(4):245–258, 2008

Egan SJ, Wade TD, Shafran R, et al: Cognitive-Behavioral Treatment of Perfectionism. New York, Guilford, 2014

Enero C, Soler A, Ramos I, et al: 2783–Distress level and treatment outcome in obsessive-compulsive personality disorder (OCPD). European Psychiatry 28(1):1, 2013

Fairburn CG, Cooper Z, Shafran R: Cognitive behaviour therapy for eating disorders: a "transdiagnostic" theory and treatment. Behav Res Ther 41(5):509–528, 2003 12711261

Fiore D, Dimaggio G, Nicoló G, et al: Metacognitive interpersonal therapy in a case of obsessive-compulsive and avoidant personality disorders. J Clin Psychol 64(2):168–180, 2008 18186113

First MB: Structured Clinical Interview for DSM-IV Axis II Personality Disorders (SCID-II). Washington, DC, American Psychiatric Press, 1997

First MB, Spitzer RL, Gibbon M, et al: Structured Clinical Interview for DSM-IV Axis I Disorders–Patient Edition (SCID-I/P, Version 2.0). New York, Biometrics Research Department, New York State Psychiatric Institute, 1996

Gratz KL, Roemer L: Multidimensional assessment of emotion regulation and dysregulation: development, factor structure, and initial validation of the Difficulties in Emotion Regulation Scale. J Psychopathol Behav Assess 26:41–54, 2004

Haring M, Hewitt PL, Flett GL: Perfectionism, coping, and quality of intimate relationships. J Marriage Fam 65:143–158, 2003

Hewitt PL, Newton J, Flett GL, et al: Perfectionism and suicide ideation in adolescent psychiatric patients. J Abnorm Child Psychol 25(2):95–101, 1997 9109026

Hopwood CJ, Pincus AL, DeMoor RM, et al: Psychometric characteristics of the Inventory of Interpersonal Problems-Short Circumplex (IIP-SC) with college students. J Pers Assess 90(6):615–618, 2008 18925504

Koutoufa I, Furnham A: Mental health literacy and obsessive-compulsive personality disorder. Psychiatry Res 215(1):223–228, 2014 24262666

Kyrios M: A cognitive-behavioral approach to the understanding and management of obsessive-compulsive personality disorder, in Cognitive Psychotherapy of Psychotic and Personality Disorders: Handbook of Theory and Practice. Edited by Perris C, McGorry PD. New York, Wiley, 1998, pp 351–378

Lynch TR: Radically Open Dialectical Behavior Therapy: Theory and Practice for Treating Disorders of Overcontrol. Oakland, CA, New Harbinger Publications, 2018

Lynch TR, Cheavens JS: Dialectical behavior therapy for comorbid personality disorders. J Clin Psychol 64(2):154–167, 2008 18186120

Millon T: Disorders of Personality: DSM-III, Axis II. New York, Wiley, 1981

Ng RM: Cognitive therapy for obsessive-compulsive personality disorder— pilot study in Hong Kong Chinese patients. Hong Kong Journal of Psychiatry 15(2):50, 2005

Ost LG: Efficacy of the third wave of behavioral therapies: a systematic review and meta-analysis. Behav Res Ther 46(3):296–321, 2008 18258216

Pinto A, Ansell EB, Wright AGC: A new approach to the assessment of obsessive compulsive personality. Integrated paper session conducted at the annual meeting of the Society for Personality Assessment, Cambridge, MA, March 2011

Pinto A, Steinglass JE, Greene AL, et al: Capacity to delay reward differentiates obsessive-compulsive disorder and obsessive-compulsive personality disorder. Biol Psychiatry 75(8):653–659, 2014 24199665

Pollak JM: Obsessive-compulsive personality: theoretical and clinical perspectives and recent research findings. J Pers Disord 1(3):248–262, 1987

Rice KG, Aldea MA: State dependence and trait stability of perfectionism: a short-term longitudinal study. J Couns Psychol 53:205–212, 2006

Riley C, Lee M, Cooper Z, et al: A randomised controlled trial of cognitive-behaviour therapy for clinical perfectionism: a preliminary study. Behav Res Ther 45(9):2221–2231, 2007 17275781

Sansone RA, Hendricks CM, Sellbom M, et al: Anxiety symptoms and healthcare utilization among a sample of outpatients in an internal medicine clinic. Int J Psychiatry Med 33(2):133–139, 2003 12968826

Shafran R, Cooper Z, Fairburn CG: Clinical perfectionism: a cognitive-behavioural analysis. Behav Res Ther 40(7):773–791, 2002 12074372

Shafran R, Egan S, Wade T: Overcoming Perfectionism: A Self-Help Guide Using Cognitive Behavioral Techniques. London, Robinson (Little, Brown Book Group), 2010

Soeteman DI, Hakkaart-van Roijen L, Verheul R, et al: The economic burden of personality disorders in mental health care. J Clin Psychiatry 69(2):259–265, 2008 18363454

Sperry L: Handbook of Diagnosis and Treatment of DSM-IV-TR Personality Disorders, 2nd Edition. New York, Brunner-Routledge, 2003

Strauss JL, Hayes AM, Johnson SL, et al: Early alliance, alliance ruptures, and symptom change in a nonrandomized trial of cognitive therapy for avoidant and obsessive-compulsive personality disorders. J Consult Clin Psychol 74(2):337–345, 2006 16649878

Svartberg M, Stiles TC, Seltzer MH: Randomized, controlled trial of the effectiveness of short-term dynamic psychotherapy and cognitive therapy for Cluster C personality disorders. Am J Psychiatry 161(5):810–817, 2004 15121645

Villemarette-Pittman NR, Stanford MS, Greve KW, et al: Obsessive-compulsive personality disorder and behavioral disinhibition. J Psychol 138(1):5–22, 2004 15098711

Weissman MM, Bothwell S: Assessment of social adjustment by patient self-report. Arch Gen Psychiatry 33(9):1111–1115, 1976 962494

Wheaton MG, Pinto A: The role of experiential avoidance in obsessive-compulsive personality disorder traits. Pers Disord 8(4):383–388, 2017 27845528

Winston A, Laikin M, Pollack J, et al: Short-term psychotherapy of personality disorders. Am J Psychiatry 151(2):190–194, 1994 8296887

Young JE: Cognitive Therapy for Personality Disorders: A Schema-Focused Approach, 3rd Edition. Sarasota, FL, Professional Resource Press, 1999

APPENDIX

Pathological Obsessive-Compulsive Personality Scale (POPS)

Factor	Definition	Sample items
Specific traits		
Rigidity	Inflexible stance in relating to and viewing the world: stubborn insistence on one's point of view, demands that others comply, and criticism of alternative view	• I insist that others do things my way. • People tell me that I am inflexible.
Emotional overcontrol	Difficulty in accepting and expressing emotions as well as relating to the emotions of others	• It is difficult for me to relate to other people's emotions. • People have described me as being closed with my feelings.
Maladaptive perfectionism	Self-imposed pressure to complete tasks with precision and at a high standard, at the expense of efficiency and productivity	• I spend too much time on something in order to get it just right. • I am hard on myself when I am unable to complete a task to my high standards.
Reluctance to delegate	Unwillingness to let others complete tasks because of concerns they won't meet expectations or distrust of their ability to do it "correctly"	• There are few people who can meet my expectations. • I end up doing a lot of jobs myself because no one can live up to my standards.
Difficulty with change	Inability to cope with unexpected or unforeseen changes in one's schedule or routine	• It really irritates me when people don't stick to the plan. • I am easily upset by changes in my routine.
General factor		
OCP-pathology	Obsessive-compulsive personality dimension on a continuum of increasing severity and dysfunction	Includes all 49 POPS items.

POPS

The statements in the table describe attitudes, opinions, interests, feelings, and behaviors that people may experience. Place a check in the box that best describes the way you usually are. Please respond to every statement, even if you are not completely sure of your answer. Read each statement carefully, but don't spend too much time deciding on any one answer. *Note:* Do not be concerned if you find that some of the statements are similar to each other. Answer each item on its own without concern for your other answers.

Scoring the POPS

Reverse-score items 19 and 25.
Sum items (strongly disagree=1; disagree=2; slightly disagree=3; slightly agree=4; agree=5; strongly agree=6) under each factor and sum all items for overall OCP-pathology score.
 Rigidity: 4, 10, 11, 12, 13, 21, 22, 24, 26, 31, 32, 33, 34, 38, 41
 Emotional overcontrol: 3, 14, 28, 29, 30, 36, 48
 Maladaptive perfectionism: 1, 7, 9, 18, 27, 37, 39, 44, 45, 46, 47, 49
 Reluctance to delegate: 2, 8, 19 (r), 20, 25 (r), 35, 40, 42
 Difficulty with change: 5, 6, 15, 16, 17, 23, 39, 43
Note that item 39 is included in both the maladaptive perfectionism and difficulty with change factors.

Copyright and Permissions

Correspondence

For permission to use or adapt this instrument for clinical or research purposes, please contact
 Anthony Pinto, Ph.D.
 Northwell Health OCD Center
 Zucker Hillside Hospital
 apinto1@northwell.edu

		Strongly Disagree	Disagree	Slightly Disagree	Slightly Agree	Agree	Strongly Agree
1.	I get lost in the details.						
2.	I never let someone else do something because they almost always do it incorrectly.						
3.	I tend to keep my emotions to myself.						
4.	When someone crosses me, I make sure to get revenge.						
5.	I hate changing my plans at the last minute.						
6.	I get upset when my day's schedule is disrupted.						
7.	My need to be perfect affects how much I get done.						
8.	I often have to take over others' responsibilities to make sure that the job is done right.						
9.	I spend too much time on something in order to get it just right.						
10.	I try to convince others of what I believe to be right and wrong.						
11.	People are either with me or they are against me.						

		Strongly Disagree	Disagree	Slightly Disagree	Slightly Agree	Agree	Strongly Agree
12.	I have been told I am inconsiderate of others.						
13.	I punish those who deserve it.						
14.	Expressing emotions usually leads to embarrassment.						
15.	I am easily upset by changes in my routine.						
16.	I have trouble dealing with unforeseen events.						
17.	I have trouble with last minute changes.						
18.	I often miss the deadlines I set for myself.						
19.	I trust others to carry out tasks competently.						
20.	I tend to take on more tasks because counting on others is useless.						
21.	Other people say that I am argumentative.						
22.	I get angry when others try to change my mind.						
23.	I have difficulty adapting to change.						
24.	Others say that I am closed minded.						
25.	I am happy to let others help me in my work.						
26.	I am a stubborn person.						

		Strongly Disagree	Disagree	Slightly Disagree	Slightly Agree	Agree	Strongly Agree
27.	I often spend too much time getting organized.						
28.	I rarely feel comfortable showing affection toward others.						
29.	I hold back my feelings.						
30.	It is difficult for me to show my feelings to others.						
31.	People think I am being critical whenever I give them advice.						
32.	I insist that others do things my way.						
33.	People tell me that I am inflexible.						
34.	Others have told me I am demanding in my relationships.						
35.	When working in a group, I find that I end up doing most of the work.						
36.	People have described me as being closed with my feelings.						
37.	I will put off a task if I do not think I can do it perfectly.						
38.	People say I am critical of the way they do things.						

		Strongly Disagree	Disagree	Slightly Disagree	Slightly Agree	Agree	Strongly Agree
39.	It is hard for me to shift from one task to another.						
40.	I end up doing a lot of jobs myself because no one can live up to my standards.						
41.	People say that I dismiss points of view that differ from my own.						
42.	There are few people who can meet my expectations.						
43.	It really irritates me when people don't stick to the plan.						
44.	I frequently need extensions on deadlines.						
45.	It takes longer for me to complete a task to my high standards.						
46.	I get caught up in the details no matter what I'm doing.						
47.	I put pressure on myself to get things just right.						
48.	It is difficult for me to relate to other people's emotions.						
49.	I am hard on myself when I am unable to complete a task to my high standards.						

REFERENCES FOR THE PSYCHOMETRICS OF THE POPS

Pinto A, Ansell EB, Wright AGC: A new approach to the assessment of obsessive compulsive personality. Integrated paper session conducted at the annual meeting of the Society for Personality Assessment, Cambridge, MA, March 2011

Sadri SK, McEvoy PM, Pinto A, et al: A psychometric examination of the Pathological Obsessive Compulsive Personality Scale (POPS): initial study in an undergraduate sample. Journal of Personality Assessment 1:1–10, 2018

Wheaton MG, Pinto A: The role of experiential avoidance in obsessive-compulsive personality disorder traits. Personality Disorders: Theory, Research, and Treatment 8:383–388, 2017

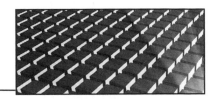

CHAPTER 10

PHARMACOLOGICAL TREATMENT OF OCPD

D. Ashkawn Ehsan, M.D.

Jon E. Grant, M.D., M.P.H., J.D.

Case Vignette

Eric, a 24-year-old male medical student, presents to your outpatient practice at the request of his significant other, Ben. Eric is in his third year of medical school and vaguely reports that things are going well. He denies any need for psychiatric services but claims Ben threatened to end their relationship if he did not seek help. On further questioning, Eric reports that he has always been a perfectionist in everything he does and attributes his success in life to his "type A personality." When asked about his academic performance, he reports a recent decline in his grades as a result of turning several papers in late and running out of time on exams. He reports having to reread and rewrite his papers multiple times before turning them in to make sure they are "perfect." Eric claims, "I'd rather turn in a perfect paper late than a flawed one on time." He often runs out of time on exams because he rereads questions and rechecks his answers several times. He goes on to report having difficulty delegating work in group projects because "no one can do the work as well as I can." He refuses to throw away his notes and past assignments, claiming, "You just never know when you'll need them again." He rarely engages in leisure activities with friends anymore because he finds this a waste of time and claims he has more important things to do. Ben, Eric's partner of 3 years, who is present during the visit, states that Eric has become more controlling recently. Ben claims, "He has to do everything himself because he doesn't think I will do it right." Ben is finding it harder and harder to live with him. Eric reports having tried therapy in the past but found it unhelpful because the therapist did not "get" him. He claims he does not currently have time for therapy and inquires about medication options for his symptoms. What do you do?

Although obsessive-compulsive personality disorder (OCPD) is the most prevalent personality disorder in the general population (Grant et al. 2012), no medications have been approved by the U.S. Food and Drug Administration for the treatment of OCPD (Ripoll et al. 2011), and only one randomized controlled trial (RCT) of drug treatment for OCPD exists (Ansseau 2000). Even with a limited evidence base for treatment, many providers have used serotonin reuptake inhibitors (SRIs) for the treatment of OCPD or OCPD traits on the basis of a possible relationship between OCPD and obsessive-compulsive disorder (OCD) (for a detailed comparison between the two disorders, see Chapter 3, "OCPD and Its Relationship to Obsessive-Compulsive and Hoarding Disorders"). In this chapter, we summarize the existing data on the pharmacological treatment of OCPD. These data include a case report, an open-label study, and an RCT examining the effects of various medications on OCPD diagnosis and traits as a primary outcome (Table 10–1), as well as various other studies, including RCTs, examining medication effects on OCPD diagnosis and traits as a secondary outcome in other psychiatric disorders (Table 10–2).

SELECTIVE SEROTONIN REUPTAKE INHIBITORS

Selective serotonin reuptake inhibitors (SSRIs) are by far the most studied class of psychotropic medications in the treatment of OCPD, as they are in the treatment of OCD. Because SSRIs have been shown to be the most efficacious medication class in treating patients with OCD (Hirschtritt et al. 2017), many clinicians have hypothesized that SSRIs could be helpful in patients with OCPD, assuming that the disorders have the same underlying neurobiological mechanism. Additionally, given that OCPD falls in the Cluster C personality disorders category,

TABLE 10–1. Medication trials and case reports for OCPD diagnosis and traits in a primary diagnosis of OCPD

Study	Study type	OCPD diagnosis or trait	N	Mean age	Sex	Drug dosage	Other drugs	Duration of treatment	Outcome measure	Outcome
Ansseau 2000	Randomized, double-blind, placebo-controlled trial	OCPD trait severity	24	Mean age 44.3 (±11.7)	M=15 F=9	Fluvoxamine (n=12) 50 mg/day×1 week, then 100 mg/day×11 weeks; placebo (n=12)	No	3 months	DSM-III-R OCPD features rated on 5-point scale (0=absent, 4=very severe) for total severity score	Mean total score change: 18.6–13.7, t=4.39, P=0.0003
Ansseau 1994	Open-label trial	OCPD trait severity	4	Mean age 43.7 (±6.5)	M=4 F=0	Fluvoxamine 50 mg/day× 1 week, then 100 mg/day for remainder of study	No	3 months	DSM-III-R OCPD features rated on 5-point scale (0=absent, 4=very severe) for total severity score	Mean total score change: 16.2 (±2.9)–11.7 (±3.6), t=7.0, P=0.006
Greve and Adams 2002	Case report	Aggression in OCPD	1	61	M	Carbamazepine 200 mg/day × 4 weeks, then 400 mg/day× 4 weeks	No	2 months	Patient report	Patient felt considerably calmer and less likely to "fly off the handle"

TABLE 10–2. Medication trials and case reports for OCPD diagnosis and traits in other psychiatric disorders

Study	Study type	Comorbid psychiatric disorder	OCPD diagnosis or trait	N	Age (SD)	Sex	Drug	Other drugs	Duration of treatment	Outcome measure	Outcome
Saxena and Sumner 2014	Open-label trial	Hoarding disorder	OCPD trait (hoarding)	24	Mean age 51.8 (±8.1)	M=3 F=21	Venlafaxine XR mean dosage 204 mg/day (±72 mg/day)	No	12 weeks	SI-R; UHSS	Mean SI-R score significantly decreased by 32% $Z=-4.02$, $P<0.001$; mean UHSS score significantly decreased by 36% $Z=-4.20$, $P<0.0001$

TABLE 10–2. Medication trials and case reports for OCPD diagnosis and traits in other psychiatric disorders *(continued)*

Study	Study type	Comorbid psychiatric disorder	OCPD diagnosis or trait	N	Age (SD)	Sex	Drug	Other drugs	Duration of treatment	Outcome measure	Outcome
Ekselius and von Knorring 1998	RDBPGT	MDD	OCPD diagnosis	308	Sertraline: mean age 47.3 (±13.3) Citalopram: mean age 48.1 (±12.0)	Sertraline: M=40 F=105 Citalopram: M=47 F=116	Sertraline (n=145): mean dosage 82.4 mg/day Citalopram (n=163): mean dosage 33.9 mg/day	No	24 weeks	SCID	Significant reduction in number of OCPD criteria in groups; citalopram>sertraline t=2.30, P<0.05

TABLE 10–2. Medication trials and case reports for OCPD diagnosis and traits in other psychiatric disorders *(continued)*

Study	Study type	Comorbid psychiatric disorder	OCPD diagnosis or trait	N	Age (SD)	Sex	Drug	Other drugs	Duration of treatment	Outcome measure	Outcome
Mavissakalian et al. 1990	Double-blind vs. open-label trial	OCD	OCPD diagnosis	27	Mean age 33.6 (±9.5)	M=33% F=67%	Clomipramine mean dosage 253.7 mg/day (±45.8 mg/day)	N/A	12 weeks	PDQ	13% reduction in compulsive personality diagnosis (significant), 19% reduction in indecisiveness trait (substantial), and 11% reduction in perfectionism trait

TABLE 10–2. Medication trials and case reports for OCPD diagnosis and traits in other psychiatric disorders *(continued)*

Study	Study type	Comorbid psychiatric disorder	OCPD diagnosis or trait	N	Age (SD)	Sex	Drug	Other drugs	Duration of treatment	Outcome measure	Outcome
Attia et al. 1998	RDBPCT	Anorexia nervosa	OCPD traits	47	Mean age 26.2 (±7.4)	M=0 F=31	Fluoxetine (n=31): mean dosage 56 mg/day (±11.2 mg/day)±therapy Placebo (n=16): mean dosage 58.7 mg/day (±5 mg/day)+therapy	N/A	Fluoxetine: 36.1 days (±14.1 days); placebo: 37.4 days (±13.8)	SCL-90-OCS	Significant reduction in SCL-90-OCS scores from 2.5 to 1.9 $P<0.05$ in fluoxetine group; however, no significant difference compared with placebo

TABLE 10–2. Medication trials and case reports for OCPD diagnosis and traits in other psychiatric disorders *(continued)*

Study	Study type	Comorbid psychiatric disorder	OCPD diagnosis or trait	N	Age (SD)	Sex	Drug	Other drugs	Duration of treatment	Outcome measure	Outcome
Santonastaso et al. 2001	Open-label, controlled trial	Anorexia nervosa	OCPD trait (perfectionism)	22	Mean age 19.0 (±3.2)	N/A	Sertraline ($n=11$): mean dosage 68.2 mg/day+therapy Control group ($n=11$): therapy only	No	Sertraline: 100.9 days (±14.1 days); control group: 102.9 (±10.3)	EDI-P	Significant reduction in EDI-P scores in sertraline group $P<0.005$; sertraline>control $F(1,20)=4.93$, $P<0.05$
Nickel et al. 2006	RDBPCT	Borderline personality disorder	OCPD traits	52	Mean age: aripiprazole 22.1 (±3.4) placebo 21.2 (±4.6)	Aripiprazole M=5 F=21 Placebo M=4 F=22	Aripiprazole ($n=26$) 15 mg/day Matching placebo ($n=26$)	No	8 weeks	SCL-90-R-OCS	Significant reduction in SCL-90-R-OCS score in aripiprazole group compared with placebo group, $P=0.01$

TABLE 10–2. Medication trials and case reports for OCPD diagnosis and traits in other psychiatric disorders *(continued)*

Study	Study type	Comorbid psychiatric disorder	OCPD diagnosis or trait	N	Age (SD)	Sex	Drug	Other drugs	Duration of treatment	Outcome measure	Outcome
Goldberg et al. 1986	RDBPCT	Borderline and schizotypal personality disorders	OCPD traits	50	Mean age 32	M=42% F=58%	Thiothixene ($n=24$) mean dosage 8.7 mg/day Placebo ($n=26$) mean dosage 26.4 mg	No	12 weeks	SLC-90-OCS	Greater improvement in SLC-90-OCS scores in thiothixene group compared with placebo but not statistically significant
Fava et al. 1994	Open-label trial	MDD	OCPD trait (perfectionism)	67	Mean age 38.1 (±11.5)	M=14 F=53	Fluoxetine 20 mg/day	No	8 weeks	DAS	Significant reduction in mean DAS scores: 145.25 (±39.90)–132.36 (±34.32), $t(65)=4.0$, $P<0.0002$

TABLE 10–2. Medication trials and case reports for OCPD diagnosis and traits in other psychiatric disorders *(continued)*

Study	Study type	Comorbid psychiatric disorder	OCPD diagnosis or trait	N	Age (SD)	Sex	Drug	Other drugs	Duration of treatment	Outcome measure	Outcome
Peselow et al. 1990	RDBPCT	MDD	OCPD trait (perfectionism)	112	Age range 18–65	N/A	Antidepressant group (n=77), fluoxetine 20–60 mg/day, clovoxamine 50–350 mg/day, and imipramine 70–245 mg/day Placebo group (n=35)	N/A	3–6 weeks	DAS	Reduction in DAS scores in antidepressant group responders no different than that in placebo group responders

TABLE 10–2. Medication trials and case reports for OCPD diagnosis and traits in other psychiatric disorders *(continued)*

Study	Study type	Comorbid psychiatric disorder	OCPD diagnosis or trait	N	Age (SD)	Sex	Drug	Other drugs	Duration of treatment	Outcome measure	Outcome
Saxena et al. 2007	Open-label trial	OCD	OCPD trait (hoarding)	79	Hoarders ($n=32$): mean age 48.7 (±9.7); non-hoarders ($n=47$): mean age 32.7 (±7.9)	Hoarders: M=9 F=23 Non-hoarders: M=32 F=15	Paroxetine mean dosage 41.6 mg/day (±12.8 mg/day)	No	80.4 days (±23.5 days)	UHSS	Significant reduction in UHSS scores in hoarders, $F(24.58)$, df=1,16, $P<0.001$
Popa et al. 2013	Open-label trial	Generalized anxiety disorder	Agreeableness in OCPD	31	Mean age 36.10	M=14 F=17	Escitalopram 10 mg/day	N/A	6 months	DECAS	Increase in "agreeableness" personality dimension scores $t=-2.72$, df=30, two-tailed 0.000, $P<0.01$

TABLE 10–2. Medication trials and case reports for OCPD diagnosis and traits in other psychiatric disorders *(continued)*

Study	Study type	Comorbid psychiatric disorder	OCPD diagnosis or trait	N	Age (SD)	Sex	Drug	Other drugs	Duration of treatment	Outcome measure	Outcome
Stein et al. 1997	Case series n=5	Bipolar disorder, Alzheimer's dementia	OCPD trait (hoarding)	1	61	F	Haloperidol 15 mg/day + thioridazine 100 mg/day + carbamazepine 400 mg/day	N/A	4 weeks	CGI	CGI=2 (much improved)
		Schizophrenia, Alzheimer's dementia	OCPD trait (hoarding)	1	69	M	Haloperidol 20 mg/day + thioridazine 200 mg/day	N/A	4 months	CGI	CGI=2 (much improved)
		Schizophrenia, Alzheimer's dementia	OCPD trait (hoarding)	1	68	F	Thioridazine 350 mg/day	N/A	2 months	CGI	CGI=3 (minimally improved)
		Schizophrenia, Alzheimer's dementia	OCPD trait (hoarding)	1	57	F	Haloperidol 10 mg/day + thioridazine 100 mg/day	N/A	4 months	CGI	CGI=2 (much improved)

TABLE 10–2. Medication trials and case reports for OCPD diagnosis and traits in other psychiatric disorders *(continued)*

Study	Study type	Comorbid psychiatric disorder	OCPD diagnosis or trait	N	Age (SD)	Sex	Drug	Other drugs	Duration of treatment	Outcome measure	Outcome
		Schizophrenia, Alzheimer's dementia	OCPD trait (hoarding)	1	62	F	Haloperidol 1 mg/day + thioridazine 25 mg/day	N/A	4 weeks	CGI	CGI=3 (minimally improved)
Garland and Weiss 1996	Case series *n*=8	Eczema	OCPD traits	1	11	F	Clomipramine 25–50 mg/day	No	1–4 years	Parent report	Improvement in rigidity, perfectionism, "obsessive irritability"
		Insomnia, migraines, generalized anxiety disorder	OCPD traits	1	11	F	Clomipramine 50 mg/day	No	1–4 years	Parent report	Improvement in rigidity, perfectionism, "obsessive irritability"

TABLE 10–2. Medication trials and case reports for OCPD diagnosis and traits in other psychiatric disorders *(continued)*

Study	Study type	Comorbid psychiatric disorder	OCPD diagnosis or trait	N	Age (SD)	Sex	Drug	Other drugs	Duration of treatment	Outcome measure	Outcome
		Insomnia, mild oppositional defiant disorder	OCPD traits	1	11	M	Clomipramine 25 mg/day	No	1–4 years	Parent report	Improvement in rigidity, perfectionism, "obsessive irritability"
		Panic disorder	OCPD traits	1	11	M	Clomipramine 50 mg/day	No	1–4 years	Parent report	Improvement in rigidity, perfectionism, "obsessive irritability"
		Adjustment disorder with depressed mood	OCPD traits	1	10	F	Clomipramine 75 mg/day	No	1–4 years	Parent report	Improvement in rigidity, perfectionism, "obsessive irritability"

TABLE 10–2. Medication trials and case reports for OCPD diagnosis and traits in other psychiatric disorders *(continued)*

Study	Study type	Comorbid psychiatric disorder	OCPD diagnosis or trait	N	Age (SD)	Sex	Drug	Other drugs	Duration of treatment	Outcome measure	Outcome
		Vomiting, migraines	OCPD traits	1	10	M	Paroxetine 10 mg/day	No	1–4 years	Parent report	Improvement in rigidity, perfectionism, "obsessive irritability"
		Insomnia, attention deficit disorder, whiny	OCPD traits	1	10	M	Clomipramine 10–25 mg/day + paroxetine 10 mg/day	No	1–4 years	Parent report	Improvement in rigidity, perfectionism, "obsessive irritability"
		Dysthymic disorder	OCPD traits	1	12	F	Fluoxetine 10 mg/day	No	1–4 years	Parent report	Improvement in rigidity, perfectionism, "obsessive irritability"

TABLE 10–2. Medication trials and case reports for OCPD diagnosis and traits in other psychiatric disorders *(continued)*

Study	Study type	Comorbid psychiatric disorder	OCPD diagnosis or trait	N	Age (SD)	Sex	Drug	Other drugs	Duration of treatment	Outcome measure	Outcome
Seedat and Stein 2002	Case series *n*=6	OCD	OCPD trait (hoarding)	1	65	M	Citalopram 60 mg/day	No	3 months	Patient report	Good response
		OCD, alcohol dependence, panic disorder with agoraphobia	OCPD trait (hoarding)	1	38	F	Fluoxetine 40 mg/day	No	3 months	Patient report	Good response
		OCD, Tourette's disorder	OCPD trait (hoarding)	1	23	M	Haloperidol 5 mg/day	No	12 months	Patient report	No response
		OCD, Tourette's disorder	OCPD trait (hoarding)	1	49	F	Citalopram 40 mg/day	No	6 months	Patient report	Poor response
		Trichotillomania, avoidant personality disorder	OCPD trait (hoarding)	1	20	F	Citalopram 60 mg/day	No	3 months	Patient report	Good response

TABLE 10–2. Medication trials and case reports for OCPD diagnosis and traits in other psychiatric disorders *(continued)*

Study	Study type	Comorbid psychiatric disorder	OCPD diagnosis or trait	N	Age (SD)	Sex	Drug	Other drugs	Duration of treatment	Outcome measure	Outcome
		MDD	OCPD trait (hoarding)	1	43	F	Citalopram 20 mg/day	No	1 month	Patient report	Poor response
Winsberg et al. 1999	Case series *n*=18	OCD, compulsive buying	OCPD trait (hoarding)	1	54	M	Fluoxetine ≥20 mg/day[a]; sertraline ≥50 mg/day[a]; sertraline ≥50 mg/day[a]+ methylphenidate	No	8–12 weeks	Patient report	Fluoxetine: little to no response; sertraline only: little to no response; sertraline + methylphenidate: partial response
		OCD, compulsive buying, pathological gambling	OCPD trait (hoarding)	1	48	F	Sertraline ≥50 mg/day[a]	No	8–12 weeks	Patient report	Partial response

TABLE 10–2. Medication trials and case reports for OCPD diagnosis and traits in other psychiatric disorders *(continued)*

Study	Study type	Comorbid psychiatric disorder	OCPD diagnosis or trait	N	Age (SD)	Sex	Drug	Other drugs	Duration of treatment	Outcome measure	Outcome
		OCD	OCPD trait (hoarding)	1	38	M	Sertraline ≥50 mg/day[a]	No	8–12 weeks	Patient report	Partial response
		OCD, body dysmorphic disorder	OCPD trait (hoarding)	1	33	F	Fluoxetine ≥20 mg/day[a], sertraline ≥50 mg/day[a]	No	8–12 weeks	Patient report	Fluoxetine: little to no response; sertraline: partial response
		OCD	OCPD trait (hoarding)	1	42	F	Fluoxetine ≥20 mg/day[a], fluvoxamine ≥150 mg/day[a], sertraline ≥50 mg/day[a]	No	8–12 weeks	Patient report	Fluoxetine: little to no response; fluvoxamine: partial response; sertraline: partial response

TABLE 10–2. Medication trials and case reports for OCPD diagnosis and traits in other psychiatric disorders *(continued)*

Study	Study type	Comorbid psychiatric disorder	OCPD diagnosis or trait	N	Age (SD)	Sex	Drug	Other drugs	Duration of treatment	Outcome measure	Outcome
		OCD, trichotillomania, pathological gambling	OCPD trait (hoarding)	1	46	F	Sertraline ≥50 mg/day[a], fluoxetine ≥20 mg/day[a]	No	8–12 weeks	Patient report	Sertraline: partial response; fluoxetine: partial response
		OCD, compulsive buying	OCPD trait (hoarding)	1	24	F	Sertraline ≥50 mg/day[a] + buspirone; fluoxetine ≥20 mg/day[a]; paroxetine ≥40 mg/day[a]	No	8–12 weeks	Patient report	Sertraline + buspirone: partial response; fluoxetine: partial response; paroxetine: partial response

TABLE 10–2. Medication trials and case reports for OCPD diagnosis and traits in other psychiatric disorders *(continued)*

Study	Study type	Comorbid psychiatric disorder	OCPD diagnosis or trait	N	Age (SD)	Sex	Drug	Other drugs	Duration of treatment	Outcome measure	Outcome
		OCD, compulsive buying	OCPD trait (hoarding)	1	47	F	Fluvoxamine ≥150 mg/day[a]; sertraline ≥50 mg/day[a]	No	8–12 weeks	Patient report	Fluvoxamine: partial response; sertraline: little to no response
		OCD, compulsive buying	OCPD trait (hoarding)	1	54	M	Sertraline ≥50 mg/day[a]; fluoxetine ≥20 mg/day[a]; paroxetine ≥40 mg/day[a]	No	8–12 weeks	Patient report	Sertraline: little to no response; fluoxetine: partial response; paroxetine: partial response
		OCD	OCPD trait (hoarding)	1	39	M	Fluoxetine ≥20 mg/day[a]; sertraline ≥50 mg/day[a]	No	8–12 weeks	Patient report	Fluoxetine: partial response; sertraline: little to no response

TABLE 10–2. Medication trials and case reports for OCPD diagnosis and traits in other psychiatric disorders *(continued)*

Study	Study type	Comorbid psychiatric disorder	OCPD diagnosis or trait	N	Age (SD)	Sex	Drug	Other drugs	Duration of treatment	Outcome measure	Outcome
		OCD	OCPD trait (hoarding)	1	43	M	Paroxetine ≥40 mg/day[a]; fluoxetine ≥20 mg/day[a]; sertraline ≥50 mg/day[a] + buspirone	No	8–12 weeks	Patient report	Paroxetine: marked response; fluoxetine: partial response; sertraline: little to no response
		OCD, compulsive buying	OCPD trait (hoarding)	1	57	F	Sertraline ≥50 mg/day[a]	No	8–12 weeks	Patient report	Partial response
		OCD, compulsive buying	OCPD trait (hoarding)	1	52	F	Paroxetine ≥40 mg/day[a]	No	8–12 weeks	Patient report	Little to no response

TABLE 10–2. Medication trials and case reports for OCPD diagnosis and traits in other psychiatric disorders *(continued)*

Study	Study type	Comorbid psychiatric disorder	OCPD diagnosis or trait	N	Age (SD)	Sex	Drug	Other drugs	Duration of treatment	Outcome measure	Outcome
		OCD	OCPD trait (hoarding)	1	49	F	Sertraline ≥50 mg/day[a]; fluoxetine ≥20 mg/day[a]	No	8–12 weeks	Patient report	Sertraline: partial response; fluoxetine: little to no response
		OCD, trichotillomania	OCPD trait (hoarding)	1	44	M	Fluoxetine ≥20 mg/day[a]	No	8–12 weeks	Patient report	Partial response
		OCD	OCPD trait (hoarding)	1	48	M	Sertraline ≥50 mg/day[a]; paroxetine ≥40 mg/day[a] + fenfluramine; fluoxetine ≥20 mg/day[a]	No	8–12 weeks	Patient report	Sertraline: little to no response; paroxetine + fenfluramine: little to no response; fluoxetine: little to no response

TABLE 10–2. Medication trials and case reports for OCPD diagnosis and traits in other psychiatric disorders *(continued)*

Study	Study type	Comorbid psychiatric disorder	OCPD diagnosis or trait	N	Age (SD)	Sex	Drug	Other drugs	Duration of treatment	Outcome measure	Outcome
		OCD	OCPD trait (hoarding)	1	57	M	Sertraline ≥50 mg/day[a]	No	8–12 weeks	Patient report	Partial response
		OCD	OCPD trait (hoarding)	1	54	M	Sertraline ≥50 mg/day[a]	No	8–12 weeks	Patient report	Partial response

Abbreviations. CGI=Clinical Global Impressions Scale; DAS=Dysfunctional Attitudes Scale; DECAS=DECAS Personality Inventory—Deschidere (Openness), Extraversie (Extroversion), Constinciozitates (Conscientiousness), Agreabilitate (Agreeableness), Stabilitate Emotionala (Emotional Stability); EDI-P= Eating Disorder Inventory—Perfectionism; MDD=major depressive disorder; OCD=obsessive-compulsive disorder; PDQ=Personality Diagnostic Questionnaire; RDBPGT =randomized, double-blind, parallel-group trial; RDBPCT= randomized double-blind placebo-controlled trial; SCID=Structured Clinical Interview for DSM-III-R Personality Disorders screening questionnaire; SCL-90-OCS=Symptom Checklist-90 Obsessive-Compulsive Subscale; SCL-90-R-OCS=Symptom Checklist-90–Revised Obsessive-Compulsive Subscale; SI-R=Saving Inventory—Revised; UHSS=UCLA Hoarding Severity Scale.

[a]Dosages described as "at or above."

often described as the anxious and fearful category, many clinicians have used SSRIs in an effort to reduce overall anxiety in patients with OCPD. In our review of the literature, we found that six different SSRIs—fluoxetine, fluvoxamine, sertraline, paroxetine, citalopram, and escitalopram—have been examined in the treatment of OCPD.

Fluoxetine

Fluoxetine is the most investigated SSRI in the treatment of OCPD. However, all of the fluoxetine studies examined OCPD diagnosis or traits as a secondary outcome in other primary psychiatric illnesses. In a double-blind RCT of fluoxetine for anorexia nervosa, Attia et al. (1998) secondarily investigated whether fluoxetine (mean dosage 56 mg/day±11.2 mg/day) in combination with psychotherapy for an average treatment duration of 36.1 days reduced Symptom Checklist-90–Revised Obsessive-Compulsive Subscale (SCL-90-R-OCS) scores in a total of 31 participants. Although there was a significant reduction in scores of both medication and placebo groups, there was no difference between placebo and fluoxetine groups on comparison.

Peselow et al. (1990) conducted three double-blind RCTs of antidepressants for major depressive disorder over a 4-year period. Two of these studies were a comparison of fluoxetine (dosage range 20–60 mg/day) and placebo, and one was a comparison of clovoxamine (dosage range 50–350 mg/day), imipramine (dosage range 70–245 mg/day), and placebo. The researchers later secondarily investigated whether these antidepressants reduced perfectionism scores (using the Dysfunctional Attitudes Scale [DAS]) and found no difference between the 41 antidepressant group responders (which included participants from the fluoxetine, clovoxamine, and imipramine groups) and the 11 placebo group responders after 3–6 weeks of treatment. To our knowledge, clovoxamine was an investigative serotonin-norepinephrine reuptake inhibitor (SNRI) that was never marketed but was studied in the treatment of depression and anxiety between the 1970s and 1990s. In an open-label trial of fluoxetine for major depressive disorder, Fava et al. (1994) reported a significant reduction of DAS perfectionism scores in 67 participants after 8 weeks of treatment with fluoxetine 20 mg/day.

In a case series, Winsberg et al. (1999) reported the drug treatment responses of 18 patients with OCD with hoarding (prior to DSM-5 [American Psychiatric Association 2013], hoarding was seen only as a symptom of OCPD). Responses to drug treatment were categorized on the basis of the patients' reported decrease in hoarding behavior as "marked," "partial," or "little to none." The patients participated in 8- to 12-week trials of one or more of the following medications: fluoxetine (≥20 mg/day), fluvoxamine (≥150 mg/day), sertraline (≥50 mg/day), paroxetine (≥40 mg/day), or clomipramine (≥150 mg/day). Of the 11 patients in the fluoxetine trials (≥20 mg/day), 6 patients reported partial response to fluoxetine and 5 reported little to no response.

In a case series of 6 patients, in which only 1 received a trial of fluoxetine (40 mg/day), Seedat and Stein (2002) reported that the patient, who was diagnosed with OCD, reported improvement in hoarding severity. Additionally, in a case series by Garland and Weiss (1996), 8 children with "obsessive difficult temperament" (which, as described by Garland and Weiss, is a syndrome that includes perfectionism as an essential feature) were prescribed medications for various psychiatric disorders and other somatic symptoms. The breakdown of medication trials included one of fluoxetine (10 mg/day), one of paroxetine (10 mg/day), five of clomipramine (dosage range 25–75 mg/day), and one of a combination of paroxetine (10 mg/day) and clomipramine (10–25 mg/day). Duration of treatment was reported as 1–4 years. All 8 children were noted by parents to have improvement in symptoms of "obsessive difficult temperament," including rigidity, perfectionism, and "obsessive irritability."

Taken together, these case reports create a mixed picture of the possible efficacy of fluoxetine for OCPD traits. The literature on fluoxetine is limited by comorbidity confounders, lack of a controlled trial in OCPD without co-occurring disorders, and difficulty in choosing an appropriate subdomain of OCPD traits that might best respond to fluoxetine. In summary, these results suggest that low dosages of fluoxetine may be helpful in reducing perfectionism and hoarding in adults, as well as perfectionism, rigidity, and irritability in children.

Fluvoxamine

Although we found only three published studies of fluvoxamine, two of the studies directly examined the effect of fluvoxamine on participants with a primary diagnosis of OCPD, and one of these was a double-blind RCT (Ansseau 2000). In an initial 3-month, open-label pilot trial of fluvoxamine (50–100 mg/day) in 4 participants with DSM-III-R OCPD, Ansseau (1994) reported a statistically significant reduction in OCPD severity scores. This initial study was followed by a 3-month, double-blind, placebo-controlled study of 24 participants with DSM-IV OCPD (Ansseau 2000). Participants were evenly distributed between the medication group (fluvoxamine 50–100 mg/day) and the placebo group. The study found that fluvoxamine was superior to placebo in reducing OCPD severity. In both studies, the authors assessed OCPD severity using a scale created specifically for the study, which rated the severity of each of the eight diagnostic criteria of DSM-III-R OCPD and each of the nine diagnostic criteria of DSM-IV OCPD on a 5-point scale, ranging from 0 = absent to 4 = very severe.

In addition, in a case series, Winsberg et al. (1999) reported that 2 patients with OCD with hoarding had a partial response to fluvoxamine

($\geq$150 mg/day) with regard to hoarding severity. Although the data are limited, fluvoxamine may be a useful agent in the treatment of OCPD. The two Ansseau studies (Ansseau 1994, 2000) suggest that a low dosage of fluvoxamine (50–100 mg/day) may reduce multiple traits of OCPD instead of only a specific one such as hoarding or perfectionism. The enthusiasm for fluvoxamine, however, must be tempered by the fact that there is only a single double-blind study and it used a scale that has not been validated for assessing change in OCPD symptoms.

Sertraline

Sertraline has been examined in OCPD but only when OCPD was co-occurring with another primary psychiatric disorder. Ekselius and von Knorring (1998) conducted a 24-week randomized double-blind parallel-group study comparing sertraline (mean dosage 82.4 mg/day) with citalopram (mean dosage 33.9 mg/day) in 308 participants with major depressive disorder, 71 of whom also met criteria for OCPD. Within the OCPD subgroup of participants, both medications significantly reduced the number of OCPD criteria; however, on comparison of each medication group, sertraline was found to be inferior to citalopram in reducing the number of OCPD criteria. The Structured Clinical Interview for DSM-III-R Personality Disorders (SCID) screening questionnaire was used to assess OCPD criteria.

In an open-label controlled trial, Santonastaso et al. (2001) examined sertraline (mean dosage 68.2 mg) in combination with psychotherapy for perfectionism in 11 participants with anorexia nervosa and found that sertraline was superior to psychotherapy only (control group) in reducing scores on the Eating Disorder Inventory—Perfectionism scale (EDI-P). Average duration of treatment was 100.9 days.

Finally, Winsberg et al. (1999) reported 17 trials of sertraline ($\geq$50 mg/day) for hoarding in 16 patients with OCD. Ten patients reported partial response to sertraline (including 1 who received a combination of sertraline with an unknown dosage of buspirone), whereas 5 patients reported little to no response to the medication (including another patient who received a combination of sertraline with an unknown dosage of buspirone). One patient had two separate medication trials of sertraline, one of which was in combination with an unknown dosage of methylphenidate. This patient reported partial response to the sertraline and methylphenidate combination but little to no response to sertraline alone.

The data for sertraline, just as for the other SSRIs, are limited and mixed. The variation in dosages used in different studies could have contributed to these results; Ekselius and von Knorring (1998) and Santonastaso et al. (2001) used rather low dosages of sertraline, and Winsberg et al. (1999) reported dosages vaguely. In summary, sertraline may be helpful in reducing severity of OCPD traits, including perfectionism and hoarding.

Paroxetine

Paroxetine is less studied than the SSRIs discussed above. Saxena et al. (2007) examined paroxetine in an open-label trial of 79 participants with OCD; a subgroup of 32 participants had a diagnosis of compulsive hoarding syndrome. In 19 of these 32 participants, the UCLA Hoarding Severity Scale (UHSS) was used to quantify hoarding severity before and after an average of 80.4 days of treatment with paroxetine (mean dosage 41.6 mg/day ± 12.8 mg/day). There was a significant reduction in scores following treatment.

Winsberg et al. (1999) reported 5 cases in which paroxetine (≥40 mg/day) was used in treating OCD patients with hoarding. Of these 5 cases, 1 patient reported a marked response, 2 reported a partial response, and 2 (one of whom was treated with a combination of paroxetine and an unknown dosage of fenfluramine) reported little to no response in hoarding behavior after 8–12 weeks of treatment with paroxetine.

Last, in a case series of children with obsessive difficult temperament (a syndrome that Garland and Weiss [1996] described as including perfectionism as an essential feature), parents of 2 children reported improvement in rigidity, perfectionism, and obsessive irritability following treatment with paroxetine (1 child with paroxetine 10 mg/day and the other with a combination of paroxetine 10 mg/day and clomipramine 10–25 mg/day). Duration of treatment was between 1 and 4 years.

Although the information for paroxetine is limited and mixed, it is worth mentioning that paroxetine was the only medication in the case series by Winsberg et al. (1999) to have a marked response on hoarding. These results suggest that paroxetine at high dosages (≥40 mg/day) might be helpful in the treatment of hoarding in adults with OCPD and at low dosages (10 mg/day) might be beneficial in children for the treatment of rigidity, perfectionism, and irritability due to OCPD.

Citalopram

Although there are limited data examining the use of citalopram in OCPD compared with other SSRIs, there is some evidence supporting its superiority to sertraline. In the 24-week randomized double-blind parallel-group study mentioned previously, Ekselius and von Knorring (1998) found citalopram (mean dosage 33.9 mg/day) to be superior to sertraline (82.4 mg/day) in reducing the number of OCPD criteria in a subgroup of 71 depressed participants with a co-occurring OCPD diagnosis. The SCID screening questionnaire was used to assess OCPD criteria.

Additionally, in a case series by Seedat and Stein (2002), 4 patients with OCD reported how their hoarding behavior responded to various dosages of citalopram. Two patients reported good response with citalopram (60 mg/day for 12 weeks), whereas the other 2 reported poor response with citalopram (one at 20 mg/day for 4 weeks and the other at 40 mg/day for 24 weeks).

The case series by Seedat and Stein (2002) presented mixed reports of improvement in hoarding behavior with citalopram, although this may be due to variations in dosage because patients taking higher dosages reported better response to the medication than patients taking lower dosages. The results of the Ekselius and von Knorring (1998) study, however, suggest that citalopram is superior to sertraline in reducing the number of overall OCPD criteria. Taken together, these results suggest that high dosages of citalopram (40–60 mg/day) are potentially helpful in reducing OCPD traits, including hoarding.

Escitalopram

Escitalopram is the least studied SSRI in the treatment of OCPD, with only a single open-label trial published. Popa et al. (2013) found a significant increase in mean scores of the personality dimension "agreeableness" in 31 participants with generalized anxiety disorder and OCPD after 6 months of treatment with escitalopram (10 mg/day). The study used the DECAS Personality Inventory, which scores each of the big five personality factors (openness, extroversion, conscientiousness, agreeableness, and emotional stability). Although agreeableness is not a criterion of OCPD, people with OCPD are often described as stubborn, and the results of this study suggested that escitalopram may be helpful in treating stubbornness in OCPD.

SEROTONIN-NOREPINEPHRINE REUPTAKE INHIBITORS

There are few existing reports of using SNRIs to treat OCPD. The lack of trials may be due to the limited use of SNRIs in the treatment of OCD; however, considering the presence of underlying anxiety in OCPD, one could expect benefit with SNRIs, which are commonly used for the treatment of anxiety disorders. Two SNRIs, venlafaxine and clovoxamine, were mentioned in studies and case reports of pharmacotherapy for OCPD.

Venlafaxine

In a single open-label trial, Saxena and Sumner (2014) reported a significant reduction in hoarding severity in 24 participants with OCPD after

12 weeks of treatment with venlafaxine XR (mean dosage 204 mg/day ± 72 mg/day). Hoarding severity was assessed using the Saving Inventory—Revised (SI-R) and the UHSS. Score reductions on both measures were significant. Venlafaxine at a low dosage may be beneficial in treating hoarding in OCPD, although results are limited to this single study.

Clovoxamine

Very little information is available about the use of clovoxamine (an investigative drug that, to our knowledge, was never marketed) in OCPD or other psychiatric disorders. As mentioned in the subsection "Fluoxetine" above, in a study of three different antidepressants for major depression, Peselow et al. (1990) secondarily investigated whether 3–6 weeks of treatment with either fluoxetine (20–60 mg/day), clovoxamine (50–350 mg/day), or imipramine (70–245 mg/day) reduced DAS perfectionism scores. They found no difference between the antidepressant responder group and the placebo responder group. These results suggest that clovoxamine, regardless of its unavailability, is not effective in treating perfectionism in OCPD.

TRICYCLIC ANTIDEPRESSANTS

Limited data exist regarding the use of tricyclic antidepressants (TCAs) in OCPD despite the known efficacy of clomipramine in the treatment of OCD. Given the side-effect profile of TCAs compared with SSRIs, this limited research may not come as a surprise, especially for the treatment of a personality disorder that patients often find ego-syntonic.

Clomipramine

Clomipramine is often used as a first-line agent (in addition to SSRIs) in the treatment of OCD, which would lead one to believe that a rather robust evidence base for its use in OCPD might exist. However, there has been limited investigation of the use of clomipramine in OCPD. In a study of 27 participants with OCD, Mavissakalian et al. (1990) secondarily analyzed reduction in overall DSM-III personality disorders and personality traits over the course of 12 weeks of treatment with clomipramine (mean dosage 253.7 mg/day ± 45.8 mg/day). Using the Personality Diagnostic Questionnaire (PDQ), they found a 13% reduction in compulsive personality diagnoses, which was considered statistically significant. They also reported a 19% reduction in indecisiveness, which was considered a substantial improvement, and an 11% reduction in perfectionism. Both indecisiveness and perfectionism were considered personality traits of the compulsive personality disorder category.

Additionally, in a case series by Garland and Weiss (1996), parents reported an improvement in rigidity, perfectionism, and obsessive irritability in six children after 1–4 years of treatment with clomipramine (dosage range 10–75 mg/day; one child received clomipramine in combination with paroxetine 10 mg/day). Medications were initially prescribed for various psychiatric disorders and other somatic symptoms. These children were described as having *obsessive difficult temperament*, a syndrome described by Garland and Weiss, which included perfectionism as an essential feature. All of these results suggest that at higher dosages (≥250 mg/day), clomipramine might be helpful in reducing perfectionism and indecisiveness in adults with OCPD, whereas at lower dosages (10–75 mg/day), it might be helpful in reducing perfectionism in children.

Imipramine

Imipramine was mentioned in only a single study. As discussed in the earlier sections on fluoxetine and clovoxamine, Peselow et al. (1990) found no difference between the antidepressant responder group and the placebo responder group in the reduction of DAS perfectionism scores in participants with major depressive disorder. Participants in the antidepressant group received fluoxetine (20–60 mg/day), clovoxamine (50–350 mg/day), or imipramine (70–245 mg/day) for a total of 3–6 weeks. The results of this study suggested that imipramine is no more effective than placebo in reducing perfectionism.

ANTIPSYCHOTICS

With few existing studies examining the efficacy of antipsychotics in treating OCPD and the often intolerable side-effect profile of these medications, the use of antipsychotics for the treatment of OCPD is questionable. Although there have been studies assessing the use of antipsychotics as augmentation in the treatment of OCD, the evidence in OCPD is limited. On review, more studies were found investigating the use of first-generation antipsychotics (FGAs) than second-generation antipsychotics (SGAs).

First-Generation Antipsychotics

Although more studies have examined the use of FGAs than SGAs in treating OCPD, the data are rather mixed. In a 12-week double-blind RCT of thiothixene for borderline and schizotypal personality disorders, Goldberg and colleagues (1986) secondarily investigated whether thiothixene (mean dosage 8.7 mg/day) reduced Symptom Checklist-90 Obsessive-Compulsive Subscale (SCL-90-OCS) scores in a total of 50 participants. Although they found a greater improvement of scores in the thiothixene group, this difference was not statistically significant.

In a case series examining hoarding in five geriatric inpatients with various primary psychiatric disorders, Stein et al. (1997) rated hoarding severity using the Clinical Global Impressions Scale (CGI). One patient was rated as having much improvement in hoarding severity after 4 weeks of treatment with a combination of haloperidol (15 mg/day), thioridazine (100 mg/day), and carbamazepine (400 mg/day). A second patient was rated as having much improvement after 4 months of treatment with a combination of haloperidol (20 mg/day) and thioridazine (200 mg/day). A third patient was also rated as having much improvement after 4 months of treatment at lower dosages (haloperidol 10 mg/day and thioridazine 100 mg/day), whereas another patient was rated as having minimal improvement after 4 weeks of treatment with even lower dosages (haloperidol 1 mg/day and thioridazine 25 mg/day). Additionally, one patient was rated as having minimal improvement after 2 months of treatment with thioridazine (350 mg/day) alone.

Finally, in a case report by Seedat and Stein (2002), a patient with Tourette's disorder, OCD, and the OCPD trait of hoarding reported no improvement in hoarding severity after 1 year of treatment with haloperidol (5 mg/day). The results of all of these studies suggest limited efficacy of FGAs in the treatment of OCPD. Specifically, thiothixene was no more effective than placebo at decreasing OCPD traits. Haloperidol alone was reportedly ineffective at reducing hoarding severity; however, reports varied when haloperidol was examined at higher dosages and in combination with other medications, including thioridazine and carbamazepine. Thioridazine minimally improved hoarding severity when used alone. Taken together, these results suggest that a combination of haloperidol and thioridazine could be helpful in reducing hoarding.

Second-Generation Antipsychotics

Although SGAs have improved tolerability compared with FGAs, only one published study has assessed effects of SGAs in OCPD. In an 8-week double-blind RCT of aripiprazole for borderline personality disorder, Nickel et al. (2006) secondarily investigated whether aripiprazole (15 mg/day) reduced SCL-90-OCS scores in 26 participants and found that aripiprazole was superior to placebo at reducing scores. Although evidence for use of SGAs in OCPD is limited to a single agent in a single study, these results suggest that a low dosage of aripiprazole could potentially be helpful in reducing OCPD traits.

ANTIEPILEPTICS

Although aggression and irritability are not core features or diagnostic criteria of OCPD, many patients and loved ones of patients with OCPD commonly report these symptoms. These symptoms become particularly noticeable when individuals with OCPD experience loss of control or resistance from others. Antiepileptics have been successfully used for treatment of aggression in various psychiatric disorders and thus may have some utility in OCPD.

Carbamazepine

In a case report by Greve and Adams (2002), a patient with a primary diagnosis of OCPD reported improvement in aggression after 2 months of treatment with carbamazepine (200–400 mg/day) before the medication was discontinued because of a rash. In a case study, Stein et al. (1997) reported that the hoarding behavior of a geriatric inpatient, as assessed using the CGI, improved following treatment with a combination of haloperidol (15 mg/day), thioridazine (100 mg/day), and carbamazepine (400 mg/day) for 4 weeks. The patient had a primary diagnosis of bipolar disorder and comorbid Alzheimer's dementia. Although studies are limited, the reported findings suggest the potential for use of carbamazepine alone for treating aggression associated with OCPD and in combination with antipsychotics for the treatment of hoarding in OCPD.

SUMMARY OF FINDINGS

SSRIs are the most studied medication class in the treatment of OCPD, followed by TCAs and then SNRIs. There are many fewer studies investigating antipsychotics and fewer still examining mood stabilizers in the treatment of OCPD. Investigated SSRIs include fluvoxamine, fluoxetine, sertraline, paroxetine, citalopram, and escitalopram.

Of these drugs, fluvoxamine was the only medication used in a double-blind RCT primarily assessing OCPD trait severity as an outcome. In that trial, fluvoxamine was found to be superior to placebo at decreasing severity of multiple OCPD traits. The results should be interpreted with caution, however, because the scale used to assess OCPD severity was created specifically for the study, and therefore its validity and reliability are not established. In addition, there was a single case report of partial response in hoarding severity with fluvoxamine treatment in a patient with OCD and hoarding. Together, these results suggest that low dosages of fluvoxamine (100–150 mg/day) may be helpful in reducing severity of OCPD traits, including hoarding.

Fluoxetine appeared in the most studies but was found to be effective in reducing perfectionism in only one open-label trial. Additionally, in one case, a child's parents reported reduction of rigidity, perfectionism, and obsessional irritability with fluoxetine, and two separate case series reported mixed effects on hoarding severity. These findings suggest that both low and high dosages of fluoxetine (20–60 mg/day) could be beneficial in reducing perfectionism and hoarding in OCPD in adults, whereas low dosages (10 mg/day) might be potentially helpful in reducing rigidity, perfectionism, and irritability due to OCPD in children.

Sertraline at low dosages (<100 mg/day) was found to be superior to placebo in reducing perfectionism in a single open-label trial but inferior to citalopram in reducing OCPD criteria in a separate study. Sertraline also had some effect on hoarding in a case series, which suggests that it could reduce perfectionism and hoarding in OCPD at low dosages (50–100 mg/day).

The results of a single open-label trial and two case series suggest that paroxetine at a relatively low dosage (10–40 mg/day) might help reduce hoarding in adults with OCPD as well as rigidity, perfectionism, and irritability in children with OCPD traits. Citalopram at high dosages (40–60 mg/day) was found to be superior to sertraline in reducing overall OCPD diagnosis in participants with major depression and may also be helpful for hoarding in patients with OCD and other psychiatric disorders. Results of a single case report suggest that escitalopram at a low dosage (10 mg/day) might improve agreeableness in OCPD. Both low and high dosages of SSRIs showed some efficacy in treatment of OCPD. Aside from two reports of citalopram being more effective for hoarding at higher dosages (60 mg/day) than lower dosages, there is little evidence supporting the need for exceedingly high dosages of SSRIs in the treatment of OCPD, as often seen with the treatment of OCD.

The SNRIs examined in OCPD include venlafaxine and clovoxamine (an investigative drug that, to our knowledge, was never marketed). On the basis of the results of an open-label trial, a high dosage (>200 mg/day) of venlafaxine XR might be effective in reducing hoarding in OCPD. Clovoxamine was no more efficacious than placebo at reducing perfectionism.

The TCAs studied in OCPD include clomipramine and imipramine. The combined results of studies investigating clomipramine suggest that it may be helpful in reducing OCPD criteria in adults and OCPD traits such as perfectionism, rigidity, and irritability in children. Although higher dosages (250 mg/day) may be needed in adults, lower dosages (10–75 mg/day) may be sufficient in children. Imipramine (dosage range 70–245 mg/day), however, was no more effective than placebo in reducing perfectionism and thus lacks evidence for use in OCPD.

With regard to antipsychotics, there are more studies investigating the use of FGAs than SGAs in OCPD. Thiothixene was found to be no more effective than placebo at decreasing OCPD traits. Per results of several case reports, haloperidol may reduce hoarding when administered in combination with other drugs, including thioridazine and carbamazepine, but not when given alone. Additionally, low dosages of thioridazine alone may be effective for hoarding. In regard to SGAs, results from a single RCT suggest that a low dosage (15 mg/day) of aripiprazole might be helpful in reducing OCPD traits, particularly in patients with co-occurring borderline personality disorder.

The only mood stabilizer mentioned in the treatment of OCPD is carbamazepine, which was shown to be potentially helpful at lower dosages (400 mg/day) for aggression and hoarding in OCPD.

Returning to the case vignette about Eric from the beginning of this chapter, an SSRI would be a reasonable medication to try. Given its reported benefit in reducing multiple OCPD traits rather than a single one, fluvoxamine (50 mg/day) would be a good place to start. On the basis of study results, a high dose may not be required given that most patients showed improvement with 50–100 mg/day. Another option— also based on its effect on multiple OCPD traits rather than just one— would be citalopram (20 mg/day), with a plan to increase the dosage to 40–60 mg/day if needed and tolerated, because higher dosages were reported in studies for OCPD.

LIMITATIONS AND FUTURE DIRECTIONS

One major limitation regarding pharmacological treatment of OCPD is the lack of high-quality studies, particularly RCTs, directly assessing medication efficacy in treatment of OCPD as a primary outcome. As mentioned, the majority of existing studies have secondarily investigated effects of medications on OCPD in patients with other psychiatric disorders. This is likely partially due to long-standing controversy over experimenting on patients with personality disorders and using medications to alter personality. Another possible explanation for the lack of controlled medication trials for OCPD is a misconception that there is little demand or need for pharmacological treatment options for personality disorders. Additionally, the nature of OCPD itself can be a barrier to research because many individuals with OCPD find the traits ego-syntonic and are not particularly interested in changing their ways and/or do not see a need for treatment.

Additionally, there is no current gold standard of assessment for OCPD. Although the studies mentioned included various scales to assess severity of different OCPD traits, there is limited research in their validity and reliability. As a result of this limitation in rating scales, a majority of the studies have focused on very specific OCPD traits, including perfectionism and hoarding, because scales for these traits are the only ones that exist.

The results of studies examining the validity and reliability of several scales used in the existing trials have been summarized. Kim et al. (1992) performed a study assessing the validity and reliability of the SCL-90-OCS in patients with OCD but not OCPD. Regardless, they found the scale to be significantly less reliable when compared with the Yale-Brown Obsessive-Compulsive Scale and the National Institute of Mental Health Global Obsessive-Compulsive Scale. Overall, their findings suggest that the scale may not be a sensitive tool in assessing change in obsessive-compulsive symptoms.

In a study measuring the validity of the UHSS in patients with a diagnosis of hoarding disorder, Saxena et al. (2015) found that the scale showed internal consistency, construct validity, convergent validity, and known-groups discriminant validity. They found that the scale validly measures core symptoms, associated features, and functional impairment of patients with hoarding disorder.

Rogers and colleagues (2009) examined the psychometric properties and factor structure of the DAS in a sample of adolescents with major depressive disorder and found that the scale demonstrated high internal consistency and correlated significantly with self-report and interview-based measures of depression. These findings, however, were not replicated by Floyd et al. (2004) in a study assessing factor structure, reliability, and validity of the DAS in older adults.

Psychometric evaluation of the SI-R found that the SI-R may be valid and reliable in the measurement of hoarding disorder in older adults (Ayers et al. 2017). Frost et al. (2004) also reported high internal consistency and good test-retest reliability of the SI-R in patients with hoarding.

Future directions in the treatment of OCPD should begin with the development of a valid and reliable rating scale to assess the severity of symptoms in OCPD. Such a tool could then be used in additional studies, specifically RCTs, to assess the use of various drugs in the treatment of OCPD. Further assessment of SSRIs in a controlled method would be valuable considering that the majority of existing data suggests some benefit in the treatment of OCPD. This information would assist in creating evidence-based treatment protocols for providers caring for individuals seeking treatment for OCPD. Having treatment guidelines for OCPD would help prevent unnecessary and ineffective medication trials, which can result in unsuccessful treatment outcomes, potential worsening of symptoms, wasted resources, economic burden on society and the health care system, and most importantly, unnecessary patient exposure to psychotropic medications and associated side effects. Finally, encouraging providers to ask their patients about OCPD symptoms and provide psychoeducation on OCPD could help foster an environment that encourages patients to discuss their symptoms and lessens stigma around seeking treatment for OCPD.

TAKE-HOME POINTS

- SSRIs are the most studied medication class and carry the most evidence in the treatment of OCPD. Both low and high dosages were found to be effective in treating OCPD traits, including perfectionism and hoarding.

- Perfectionism and hoarding were the most common OCPD traits assessed in studies, and thus, focusing on these symptoms may be a good starting point for treating patients with OCPD.

- A gold standard for the assessment of OCPD severity does not currently exist, which poses major limitations in quality research. Future directions in treatment of OCPD would benefit from the development of a valid and reliable scale that can be used globally to assess OCPD severity for future studies.

REFERENCES

American Psychiatric Association: Diagnostic and Statistical Manual of Mental Disorders, 5th Edition. Arlington, VA, American Psychiatric Association, 2013

Ansseau M: Are SSRIs useful in obsessive-compulsive personality disorder? Eur Neuropsychopharmacol 4(3):266–267, 1994

Ansseau M: Serotonergic antidepressants in obsessive-compulsive personality disorder, in Obsessive-Compulsive Disorder. Edited by Maj M. New York, Wiley, 2000, pp 89–91

Attia E, Haiman C, Walsh BT, et al: Does fluoxetine augment the inpatient treatment of anorexia nervosa? Am J Psychiatry 155(4):548–551, 1998 9546003

Ayers CR, Dozier ME, Mayes TL: Psychometric evaluation of the Saving Inventory–Revised in older adults. Clin Gerontol 40(3):191–196, 2017 28452663

Ekselius L, von Knorring L: Personality disorder comorbidity with major depression and response to treatment with sertraline or citalopram. Int Clin Psychopharmacol 13(5):205–211, 1998 9817625

Fava M, Bless E, Otto MW, et al: Dysfunctional attitudes in major depression. Changes with pharmacotherapy. J Nerv Ment Dis 182(1):45–49, 1994 8277301

Floyd M, Scogin F, Chaplin WF: The Dysfunctional Attitudes Scale: factor structure, reliability, and validity with older adults. Aging Ment Health 8(2):153–160, 2004 14982720

Frost RO, Steketee G, Grisham J: Measurement of compulsive hoarding: Saving Inventory-Revised. Behav Res Ther 42(10):1163–1182, 2004 15350856

Garland EJ, Weiss M: Case study: obsessive difficult temperament and its response to serotonergic medication. J Am Acad Child Adolesc Psychiatry 35(7):916–920, 1996 8768352

Goldberg SC, Schulz SC, Schulz PM, et al: Borderline and schizotypal personality disorders treated with low-dose thiothixene vs placebo. Arch Gen Psychiatry 43(7):680–686, 1986 3521531

Grant JE, Mooney ME, Kushner MG: Prevalence, correlates, and comorbidity of DSM-IV obsessive-compulsive personality disorder: results from the National Epidemiologic Survey on Alcohol and Related Conditions. J Psychiatr Res 46(4):469–475, 2012 22257387

Greve KW, Adams D: Treatment of features of obsessive-compulsive personality disorder using carbamazepine. Psychiatry Clin Neurosci 56(2):207–208, 2002 11952927

Hirschtritt ME, Bloch MH, Mathews CA: Obsessive-compulsive disorder: advances in diagnosis and treatment. JAMA 317(13):1358–1367, 2017 28384832

Kim SW, Dysken MW, Kuskowski M: The Symptom Checklist-90: Obsessive-Compulsive subscale: a reliability and validity study. Psychiatry Res 41(1):37–44, 1992 1561287

Mavissakalian M, Hamann MS, Jones B: DSM-III personality disorders in obsessive-compulsive disorder: changes with treatment. Compr Psychiatry 31(5):432–437, 1990 2225802

Nickel MK, Muehlbacher M, Nickel C, et al: Aripiprazole in the treatment of patients with borderline personality disorder: a double-blind, placebo-controlled study. Am J Psychiatry 163(5):833–838, 2006 16648324

Peselow ED, Robins C, Block P, et al: Dysfunctional attitudes in depressed patients before and after clinical treatment and in normal control subjects. Am J Psychiatry 147(4):439–444, 1990 2180328

Popa CO, Nirestean A, Ardelean M, et al: Dimensional personality change after combined therapeutic intervention in the obsessive-compulsive personality disorders. Acta Medica Transilvanica 2(1):290–292, 2013

Ripoll LH, Triebwasser J, Siever LJ: Evidence-based pharmacotherapy for personality disorders. Int J Neuropsychopharmacol 14(9):1257–1288, 2011 21320390

Rogers GM, Park J-H, Essex MJ, et al: The dysfunctional attitudes scale: psychometric properties in depressed adolescents. J Clin Child Adolesc Psychol 38(6):781–789, 2009 20183662

Santonastaso P, Friederici S, Favaro A: Sertraline in the treatment of restricting anorexia nervosa: an open controlled trial. J Child Adolesc Psychopharmacol 11(2):143–150, 2001 11436953

Saxena S, Sumner J: Venlafaxine extended-release treatment of hoarding disorder. Int Clin Psychopharmacol 29(5):266–273, 2014 24722633

Saxena S, Brody AL, Maidment KM, et al: Paroxetine treatment of compulsive hoarding. J Psychiatr Res 41(6):481–487, 2007 16790250

Saxena S, Ayers CR, Dozier ME, et al: The UCLA Hoarding Severity Scale: development and validation. J Affect Disord 175:488–493, 2015 25681559

Seedat S, Stein DJ: Hoarding in obsessive-compulsive disorder and related disorders: a preliminary report of 15 cases. Psychiatry Clin Neurosci 56(1):17–23, 2002 11929567

Stein DJ, Laszlo B, Marais E, et al: Hoarding symptoms in patients on a geriatric psychiatry inpatient unit. S Afr Med J 87(9):1138–1140, 1997 9358832

Winsberg ME, Cassic KS, Koran LM: Hoarding in obsessive-compulsive disorder: a report of 20 cases. J Clin Psychiatry 60(9):591–597, 1999 10520977

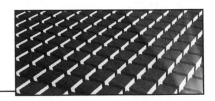

CHAPTER 11

IMPACT OF PERSONALITY DISORDERS ON PARENTING

Bekir B. Artukoglu, M.D.
Angeli Landeros-Weisenberger, M.D.
Michael H. Bloch, M.D., M.S.

Case Vignette

Stuart is a 55-year-old white male who presents for the first time to seek advice from a mental health professional. He works as regional manager in Connecticut in a real estate company that was founded by his father. Stuart's chief complaint is feeling detached from his son and daughter

Dr. Bloch and colleagues would like to thank Jessica Levine for her careful review and critiques of this manuscript prior to submission.

and being unable to love them. He is single and lives alone following his divorce 15 years earlier. He has not seen his daughter, Olivia, for more than a year and feels that his inability to show her affection may have contributed to her decision to move away from Connecticut. He meets his son, Cole, every 5–6 months for dinner but feels that their time together is far from enjoyable for either of them. Further investigation of his relationship with his children reveals that Stuart has observed a deterioration in his communication with Olivia. He describes her as having been passionate and loving as a teenager, but, to his dismay, her acts of love toward him decreased over the years, and she has barely shown him any compassion as a young adult. Stuart blames himself for being "too stiff" and "highly controlled." He feels that his personality may have pushed away his emotionally expressive daughter and may also have played a part in ending his marriage. He feels that the divorce was not all bad, however, as it allowed him to focus on "things that really matter," such as expanding his branch of the company and doing things at his own schedule. Stuart explains that his responsibilities in the company and not letting his father down mean the world to him. He admits to having spent less time with his family than his ex-wife wanted but sees this as a sacrifice to the work ethic that he inherited from his father. He is relieved that the apple didn't fall far from the tree in regard to Cole, who recently graduated from an MBA program at Yale and whom Stuart describes as being self-disciplined and orderly. However, Stuart expresses disappointment in Cole's decision to not have any children. He has found himself thinking about Cole's decision every day since Cole told him this news several weeks ago. Cole stated that it was impossible to raise children in this crazy world and insisted that this was all he had to say about the matter. Stuart worries that he may be the one to blame for Cole's decision because he was always emotionally unavailable and set a bad parental example for his son.

A personality disorder is a pervasive and inflexible pattern of inner experience and behaviors, outside of the individual's culture, that leads to distress and impairment in social, occupational, or other important areas of functioning (American Psychiatric Association 2013). Personality disorders are defined by an enduring pattern that manifests as impairments in cognition, affective states, impulse control, and interpersonal functioning. Perspectives on how to define and assess personality disorders vary greatly, so much so that the developers of DSM-5 (American Psychiatric Association 2013) opted to include two separate models for examining this group of disorders: an updated version of the traditional model (in Section II, "Diagnostic Criteria and Codes") and an alternative model that was developed by a new team (presented in Section III, "Emerging Measures and Models").

The first model groups personality disorders into three clusters based on similar characteristics, such as odd or eccentric (Cluster A, which includes paranoid, schizoid, and schizotypal personality disorders); dramatic, emotional, or erratic (Cluster B, which includes antisocial, borderline, histrionic, and narcissistic personality disorders); and anxious or fearful (Cluster C, which includes avoidant, dependent, and obsessive-compulsive personality disorders). The alternative model focuses on impairments in the four elements of personality functioning—identity, self-direction, empathy, and intimacy—and the presence of pathological personality traits from five domains—negative affectivity, detachment, antagonism, disinhibition, and psychoticism. There is a common thread to different views and models that were developed by research teams over the years: the substantial impact that personality disorder may have on self and interpersonal functioning, which in turn may influence parental capacity. Common clinical comorbidities should also be considered for the assessment of personality disorders and parental functioning.

Economic circumstances are thought to be linked to health, cognitive, and emotional outcomes in children. Research shows that young adults with personality disorders are economically disadvantaged and may face enduring lowered economic functioning (Niesten et al. 2016). Diagnostic interview data from a large survey study in the United States indicate past-year prevalence of personality disorders in adults to be 9.1% (Lenzenweger et al. 2007). Considering the high prevalence and complex presentation of personality disorders, with comorbidities and economic repercussions, it is important to assess and treat parental deficits in individuals with personality disorders.

Obsessive-compulsive personality disorder (OCPD) is one of the most common personality disorders, affecting 1%–2% of the population (Samuels et al. 2002; Torgersen et al. 2001), and prevalence has been described as being about 8% in a large epidemiological study of adults in the United States (Grant et al. 2004). OCPD is most common in males and in married and working individuals, and clinicians should consider how having a parent with OCPD can affect child development.

According to the Collaborative Longitudinal Personality Disorders Study, about 75% of individuals with OCPD also have or have had comorbid major depressive disorder at some point in their lifetime (McGlashan et al. 2000). Although OCPD is associated with less disability when compared with other personality disorders, 90% of individuals with personality disorders have moderate to severe impairment in at least one area of functioning.

Early psychoanalytic contributions correlate certain character traits—specifically, obstinacy, parsimony, and orderliness—with the anal phase of psychosexual development. Patients with OCPD are thought to have regressed from the castration anxiety associated with the oedipal phase of development to the relative safety of the anal period. Driven by a punitive superego, they employ defensive operation of the ego such as isolation of affect, intellectualization, reaction formation, undoing, and displacement. Persons with OCPD have considerable difficulty express-ing aggression and tend to be stubborn. It is theorized that as children, they did not feel sufficiently valued or loved by their parents, either be-cause the children perceived the parents as cold and distant or because the children required more reassurance and affection than other chil-dren. To patients with OCPD, anger and dependency are consciously unacceptable, so they defend against those feelings with defense mech-anisms such as reaction formation and isolation of affect. They strive for complete control over all anger and go to great lengths to demonstrate their independence and individualism (Gabbard 2014).

GOOD ENOUGH PARENTING

Defining good parenting is a complex task that has resulted in diverging approaches developed by different professional teams. These ap-proaches have several common main themes: insight (an awareness of one's role as a parent), finding a balance in meeting the child's day-to-day and long-term needs, putting the child's needs before the parent's own, fostering attachment, and balancing a consistent discipline with flexibility (Eve et al. 2014). *Good enough parenting* is a model that pro-motes remedying the deficits in parenting as they arise instead of pursu-ing perfectionism (Choate and Engstrom 2014; Dalzell-Ward 1957). A report on parenting and mental health underlines the importance of sev-eral factors for good enough parenting: a degree of selflessness to priori-tize the child's needs; willingness to deny the child's requests and tolerate the ensuing negative feelings; the ability to protect the child from adult concerns; respect for the child's developing autonomy; and the ability to exercise authority to provide the child with safety, education, and social opportunities (Royal College of Psychiatrists 2011). Finding a balance between providing the child with safety and the child's freedom to ex-ercise autonomy makes parenting a rather difficult task.

Another review of the contributions to the field of parenting and personality disorders implicates several behaviors in parental dysfunc-tion: neglecting basic needs of the child; putting the adults' needs first; chaos and lack of routine; and unwillingness to engage with support services (Kellett and Apps 2009). Expert opinion draws attention to the importance of parents being empathetic and sympathetic to vulnerabil-ity and dependence in children and being able to manage their own negative emotions and to tolerate these emotions when they arise in family members (Adshead 2015). Dysfunctional affective and cognitive patterns in people with personality disorders represent challenges for them when attempting to adhere to these principles of parenting.

Attachment theory, described in the next section, provides a framework for better understanding these conflicts because attachment is thought to play a role both in determining parenting capacity and in the development of personality disorder. Therefore, we could surmise that attachment issues will be an important etiological factor behind the presence of OCPD in both parental units and their offspring. Results from two studies support the idea that individuals diagnosed with OCPD or OCPD traits have never actually formed secure attachments (Nordahl and Stiles 1997; Perry et al. 2007). These studies propose that these individuals have received distant care and have been highly scrutinized during their childhood, resulting in adults who were unable to develop both emotionally and empathetically. These conditions will perpetuate this style of parenting and in turn affect their offspring.

For children with OCPD, the low self-esteem connected with their sense of not being valued often leads to an assumption that others would prefer not to put up with them, resulting in a perceived sense of distance between the child and his or her parent. Children often grow up with the conviction that they simply did not try hard enough, and as adults they chronically feel that they are not doing enough. As adults, their thought patterns are rigid and dogmatic, and they pay close attention to detail but lack spontaneity or flexibility, resulting in a stalemate in which the parent with OCPD cannot acknowledge that his or her child or loved one might have a different or better way to do things. The feelings inherent in intimate relationships, such as being a parent or part of a dyad, are threatening because of their potential to get disrupted, resulting in relationships that are often too controlling.

ATTACHMENT THEORY AND PARENTING CAPACITY OF PARENTS WITH PERSONALITY DISORDERS

Attachment theory is a term coined by British psychologist John Bowlby (1969) to describe the role of a parent to initially provide a sense of security and foundation from which the child may find confidence and eventually take excursions into the outside world. This model includes a measure of dependency between caregiver and care elicitor, which is especially active during times of threat. A sense of security provided by the caregiving parent leads to secure attachment, which transforms into an internal model of the young individual both as someone who can be cared for and as an effective caregiving parent (Bowlby 1969).

An insecure working model, on the other hand, leads to impaired management of threatening situations that include vulnerability, which manifests as an impairment in a variety of interpersonal relationships and dysfunctional parenting behaviors (Adshead et al. 2004). Insecure attachment styles in adulthood have been associated with personality disorders in clinical samples (Aaronson et al. 2006; Levy et al. 2005) and nonclinical samples (Meyer et al. 2004; Nickell et al. 2002). At times of threat when children require care and soothing from their caregivers, parents with personality disorders may become unavailable because of highly dysregulated affect and arousal systems (Royal College of Psychiatrists 2011). A systematic review of the literature on the link between personality disorder and parenting capacity implicates parental personality disorder as a risk factor for both impaired parenting behaviors and disturbed parent-infant interactions (Laulik et al. 2013).

OCPD is a common personality disorder, comprising lifelong patterns of behavior that may not necessarily cause distress in the patients themselves and may even be regarded as highly adaptive. OCPD traits are often associated with success in the work environment because of a typical devotion to work that may lead to high achievements; however, success in the work sphere often comes at a high price because family members often find individuals with OCPD very difficult to live with.

Children who cannot calm themselves or who never react to the disappearance of their attachment figure are assessed as insecurely attached. This trait is often interpreted by parents with OCPD as a sign of independence in their children. To evaluate how secure the attachment between the child and parent is, researchers often use the Strange Situation test developed by psychologist Mary Ainsworth in the 1960s while at Johns Hopkins University (Ainsworth and Wittig 1969).

Infants are hardwired to build attachment with a primary caregiver. However, in 1943, Johanna Haarer published *Die Deutsche Mutter und ihr Erstes Kind* (*The German Mother and Her First Child*), recommending that children be raised with as few attachments as possible and that excessive tenderness was to be avoided at all cost (Haarer 1943). One piece of advice was particularly pernicious: she urged mothers to ignore their babies' emotional needs. Her advice guided child rearing during the Third Reich. The Nazis wanted children who were tough, unemotional, and unempathetic and who had weak attachment to others, and they understood that withholding affection would support that goal.

Very little information about the specific nature of attachment in OCPD has yet been gleaned, but Haarer's recommendations have been demonstrated to be traumatizing even though they were viewed during the Nazi era as modern and "scientifically sound." Because of ethical reasons, randomized controlled research trials to study these recommendations for upbringing cannot be conducted; however, in a meta-analysis, Verhage et al. (2016) analyzed data from 4,819 individuals and confirmed that the quality of attachment is transmitted from generation to generation. The transmissive nature of the attachment issues with personality disorders can be observed in the case vignette presented earlier in the chapter. Stuart's desire to prioritize work over intimate relationships seems to be deeply related to the image he has of his father as a businessman. A similar transmission may be seen in Cole's decision not to have children of his own.

IMPACT OF PARENTAL PERSONALITY DISORDER ON CHILD DEVELOPMENT AND MENTAL HEALTH

Parental personality disorder has negative impacts on children that are both indirect (through interparental conflict and hostile family environment) and direct. Research has shown that parental personality disorder is also associated with mental health disorders in children. Observational studies of families in which children were diagnosed with conduct disorder and oppositional defiant disorder found higher rates of parental personality disorder (Frick et al. 1992). Studies in children with attention-deficit/hyperactivity disorder and in children with conduct disorder and hyperactivity have found significant associations between parental personality disorders and behavioral problems in children (Lahey et al. 1988; Nigg and Hinshaw 1998).

Studies found that people with personality disorder have high rates of dysfunctional intimate relationships, which have implications for child development. Marital conflict and dissatisfaction, as well as intimate partner violence, were associated with antisocial, borderline, and narcissistic personality disorders, as described in several studies (Holtzworth-Munroe 2000; South et al. 2008; White and Gondolf 2000). Systematic reviews also suggest that parents with personality disorders are more likely to engage in child maltreatment (Laulik et al. 2013; Petfield et al. 2015). As to the more direct effects of parental personality disorder, studies have shown higher rates of both deficient parenting and child abuse in family units in which parents have personality disorder (Famularo et al. 1992; Wiehe 2003). Some of the dysfunctional practices demonstrated by parents with personality disorder are inconsistent parental discipline, insensitive or intrusive parent-infant interactions, and low parental affection and support (Conroy et al. 2010; Crandell et al. 2003; Hobson et al. 2005; Johnson et al. 2006, 2008; Newman et al. 2007). In the clinical vignette presented earlier in this chapter, Stuart's OCPD traits such as being stiff and controlled seem to have contributed to the problems he has had in his relationship with his daughter. The marital conflict in the family was also likely a result of Stuart's OCPD because his wife was not pleased with how overinvested he was in his work.

Borderline personality disorder (BPD) is a Cluster B personality disorder that has been the most commonly examined personality disorder in the context of parent-child relationships. Studies found that mothers with BPD have difficulties in reflecting on their children's thoughts and emotions (Schacht et al. 2013), identifying their children's emotions in photographs (Elliot et al. 2014), and structuring young children's activities (Newman et al. 2007). Mothers with BPD find parenting to be highly stressful (Herr et al. 2008). Antisocial personality disorder is another Cluster B personality disorder that has been frequently associated with child maltreatment (Adshead et al. 2004; Johnson et al. 2008). Although research on parental personality disorder has focused on BPD and other Cluster B personality disorders (Laulik et al. 2013), a longitudinal study that investigated the associations of parental psychiatric disorders with child-rearing behavior did not find a significant association between parental OCPD traits and child-rearing difficulties (Johnson et al. 2008). Studies on specific personality disorders are needed to investigate the presence of parenting deficits with different types of personality disorder.

Few empirical studies compare the attachment styles of patients with BPD with those of patients with other personality disorders, or specifically with OCPD. In theory, one would expect these individuals to be on opposite ends of a spectrum because patients with BPD are thought to be impulsive, seek pleasure, and hold unorthodox opinions, whereas those with OCPD are thought to relish self-control, logic, and loyalty to established values. Both attachment styles were compared using the Reciprocal Attachment Questionnaire (RAQ), comparing measures of both patterns of attachment (angry withdrawal, compulsive caregiving, compulsive self-reliance, and compulsive care seeking) and dimensions of attachment (proximity seeking, separation protest, feared loss, availability of attachment figure, and use of attachment figure) (Aaronson et al. 2006). Parents with BPD had higher levels of lack of availability of the attachment figure, feared loss, lack of use of the attachment figure, and separation protest, as well as higher levels of angry withdrawal pattern and compulsive care-seeking pattern. Feared loss is a discriminating feature of BPD.

A large nationally representative survey on personality disorders and mental health comorbidities revealed significant comorbidities in individuals with any of the three personality disorder clusters; comorbidities were highest in individuals with Cluster B personality disorders (Lenzenweger et al. 2007). This survey revealed that 84.5% of the adults with BPD had experienced at least one Axis I disorder in the previous 12 months. Although data on specific personality disorders are inadequate, considerable comorbidity has been found between personality disorders and eating disorders, somatization disorders, mood disorders, anxiety disorders, and substance abuse (Bornstein and Gold 2008; Kaess et al. 2013; Shea et al. 1992; Westen and Harnden-Fischer 2001). Parental psychopathology has been associated with psychiatric symptoms in their offspring, and each of these comorbidities can potentially impact the child (Downey and Coyne 1990; Kendler 1996). A meta-analytic review of comorbidity of personality disorders and somatization disorder found a statistically significant association; comorbidity effect sizes were higher for antisocial, borderline, narcissistic, histrionic, avoidant, and dependent personality disorders (Bornstein and Gold 2008). Maternal somatization disorder may represent a risk factor for somatization in the child. Binge-eating and compulsive exercise were found to be increased in children of parents who exhibited core features of eating disorders (Lydecker and Grilo 2016). Studies suggest that children of parents who abuse substances are more likely to suffer maltreatment, to have emotional and behavioral problems, and to die by suicide (Forrester 2000).

The causal relationship between abusive experiences and personality disorders may be bidirectional. In this chapter that examines the impact of parental personality disorder, it is worth noting that physical and sexual abuse are thought to be strong predictors for development of personality disorders (Battle et al. 2004; Paris et al. 1994). A study that assessed self-reported history of child maltreatment in 600 patients who were diagnosed with personality disorders found high rates of abuse (73%) and neglect (82%) (Battle et al. 2004). Maladaptive parental behaviors in parents with or without psychiatric disorders were found to predict adolescent personality disorder and other psychiatric symptoms. A longitudinal study in 793 mothers and their offspring showed that children who experienced maternal verbal abuse during childhood were more than three times as likely as those who did not experience verbal abuse to have borderline, narcissistic, obsessive-compulsive, and paranoid personality disorders during adolescence or early adulthood (Johnson et al. 2001).

Personality disorders are thought to arise from the interplay of genetic and environmental risk factors—including dysfunctional child rearing and child maltreatment—both of which may be transmitted from parent to child. People with personality disorders are commonly individuals who experienced a form of abuse as children and are at risk to replicate malpractice as a parent. This may contribute to the heritability of personality disorder, which is thought to be moderate to high according to genetic studies on twins and families (Bassir Nia et al. 2018; Coolidge et al. 2001). One large multinational study on BPD attributed 42% of the variation in BPD features to genetic influences and 58% of the variation to environmental influences (Distel et al. 2008). Although it is important to understand the etiology and cyclical nature of personality disorders, clinicians should prioritize children's safety over sympathy for the parent in cases of child abuse and neglect.

ASSESSMENT AND TREATMENT OF PARENTING DEFICITS IN PEOPLE WITH PERSONALITY DISORDERS

Clinical impressions and research suggest that the prevalence of mental health disorders is high in children of parents with personality disorders and associated psychiatric comorbidities. Thorough assessment and treatment of parental deficits in people with personality disorders are essential to prevent future economic burden of mental health and to promote the healthy development and well-being of children.

Although there is evidence for the effectiveness of psychotherapeutic interventions for personality disorders (Bateman and Fonagy 2000; Levy et al. 2018; Sperry 2006), the ego-syntonic nature of personality disorders and the resulting poor adherence are significant barriers to treatment (McMurran et al. 2010). The long-standing course of these therapies may prevent the nonadherent patient from reaping the full benefits of the treatment (Sperry 2003).

Although having personality disorder does not guarantee parental deficiency, dysfunctional parenting practices may be severe in parents with personality disorder. Therefore, administering interventions to improve parenting practices should therefore be considered, along with treatments for personality disorders. Various assessments can be carried out to investigate the risk to the child, including assessments of parental mental health and mental state, parenting capacity, the child's emotional well-being, and evidence of significant harm to the child (Adshead et al. 2004). The complexity of risk assessment means that several professionals with different specialties may be involved in cases of maltreatment. Considering the manipulative behaviors common in certain personality disorders, it is important to avoid conflict between professionals. Financial problems, interparental conflict, and impairments in dyadic parent-child interaction may all limit parenting capacity and should be assessed. Parents' own experiences of abuse and neglect and their histories of dysfunctional or violent relationships may also be considered as risk factors for hostility toward their own children (Royal College of Psychiatrists 2011).

Transmission of dysfunctional parent-child attachment and relationship patterns across generations may partly explain the parenting deficits and the resulting mental health burden in the next generation. It may be helpful to address the experience and consequences of trauma in the parent's past. Interventions that aim to improve one's own and others' mental states and behaviors may aid parental capacity for empathy and distress or arousal tolerance (Fonagy 2002; Newman and Stevenson 2005). Specific parent-child interventions that include both parties may also foster sensitivity and understanding in the parent and promote a healthier parent-child relationship and security of attachment.

Although no studies have been conducted on treating parenting deficits in individuals with OCPD, current literature suggests that improvements in overall mental health and interpersonal relationships may benefit their parenting capacity. Therefore, we would recommend the same psychological and pharmacological treatments for parents with OCPD as for OCPD patients in general. Psychological interventions for OCPD in parents can specifically focus on exploring ways in which the disorder is affecting the parent-child relationship. Residential and day facilities may be good settings both to administer personality disorder interventions (Lees et al. 1999) and to observe and improve dyadic and interpartner relationships. It is therefore unfortunate that most of these communities do not implement interventions for parenting deficits or admit parents with personality disorder with their children (Adshead et al. 2004).

CONCLUSION

Significant limitations exist in personality disorder research and the effects of personality disorder on parenting. Evidence is mostly limited to studies on maternal personality disorder, and specific personality disorders have not received enough attention. Parental personality disorder often results in impairments in tolerance and nourishment of the vulnerable child, particularly in moments of parental stress and arousal. Presence of psychiatric comorbidities and substance abuse in the parent, socioeconomic circumstances, the quality of the interparental relationship, and support from the other parent are some of the factors that should also be considered as part of the assessment of parenting capacity. When parenting deficits are found, it is necessary to employ treatments for personality disorders and interventions to improve parenting skills and the parent-child dyadic relationship. Residential settings may be ideal to carry out multiple, detailed assessments and to introduce therapeutic changes to the family unit. The transmissible nature of personality disorders and the associated burden of mental illness in the next generation warrant more rigorous research and provision of services aimed at improving assessment of risk and development of evidence-based treatments for parenting deficits that are common in individuals with personality disorders.

TAKE-HOME POINTS

- Personality disorder may have a substantial impact on self and interpersonal functioning, which, in turn, may influence parental capacity.

- OCPD is one of the most common personality disorders in married and working individuals; therefore, the ramifications of parental OCPD for child development should be an important consideration for clinicians.

- Parents with personality disorder may find it difficult to adhere to principles of good parenting, such as being empathetic and sympathetic to vulnerability in children and being able to manage their own and their family members' negative emotions.

- Insecure attachment styles in individuals with personality disorders lead to impaired management of threatening situations that include vulnerability, which manifests as an impairment in a variety of interpersonal relationships and dysfunctional parenting behaviors.

- Personality disorders are thought to arise from the interplay of genetic and environmental risk factors—including dysfunctional child rearing and child maltreatment—both of which may be transmitted from parent to child. Although it is important to understand the etiology and cyclical nature of personality disorders, clinicians should prioritize children's safety over sympathy for the parent in cases of child abuse and neglect.

- When parenting deficits are found, it is necessary to employ treatments for personality disorder and interventions to improve parenting skills and the parent-child dyadic relationship.

REFERENCES

Aaronson CJ, Bender DS, Skodol AE, et al: Comparison of attachment styles in borderline personality disorder and obsessive-compulsive personality disorder. Psychiatr Q 77(1):69–80, 2006 16397756

Adshead G: Parenting and personality disorder: clinical and child protection implications. Advances in Psychiatric Treatment 21(1):15–22, 2015

Adshead G, Falkov A, Gopfert M: Personality disorder in parents: developmental perspectives and intervention, in Parental Psychiatric Disorder: Distressed Parents and Their Families, 2nd Edition. Edited by Gopfert M. Cambridge, UK, Cambridge University Press, 2004, pp 217–237

Ainsworth MDS, Wittig BA: Attachment and exploratory behavior of one-year-olds in a strange situation, in Determinants of Infant Behavior, Vol 4. Edited by Foss BM. London, Methuen, 1969, pp 111–136

American Psychiatric Association: Diagnostic and Statistical Manual of Mental Disorders, 5th Edition. Arlington, VA, American Psychiatric Association, 2013

Bassir Nia A, Eveleth MC, Gabbay JM, et al: Past, present, and future of genetic research in borderline personality disorder. Curr Opin Psychol 21:60–68, 2018 29032046

Bateman AW, Fonagy P: Effectiveness of psychotherapeutic treatment of personality disorder. Br J Psychiatry 177:138–143, 2000 11026953

Battle CL, Shea MT, Johnson DM, et al: Childhood maltreatment associated with adult personality disorders: findings from the Collaborative Longitudinal Personality Disorders Study. J Pers Disord 18(2):193–211, 2004 15176757

Bornstein RF, Gold SH: Comorbidity of personality disorders and somatization disorder: a meta-analytic review. J Psychopathol Behav Assess 30:154, 2008

Bowlby J: Attachment and Loss: Attachment. New York, Basic Books, 1969

Choate P, Engstrom S: The "good enough" parent: implications for child protection. Child Care in Practice 20(4):368–382, 2014

Conroy S, Marks MN, Schacht R, et al: The impact of maternal depression and personality disorder on early infant care. Soc Psychiatry Psychiatr Epidemiol 45(3):285–292, 2010 19466372

Coolidge FL, Thede LL, Jang KL: Heritability of personality disorders in childhood: a preliminary investigation. J Pers Disord 15(1):33–40, 2001 11236813

Crandell LE, Patrick MP, Hobson RP: "Still-face" interactions between mothers with borderline personality disorder and their 2-month-old infants. Br J Psychiatry 183:239–247, 2003 12948998

Dalzell-Ward AJ: The child and the family, by D.W. Winnicott (Tavistock Publications Ltd. 1957. Pp. 147. Price 12s. 6d.). Health Education Journal 15:203–204, 1957

Distel MA, Trull TJ, Derom CA, et al: Heritability of borderline personality disorder features is similar across three countries. Psychol Med 38(9):1219–1229, 2008 17988414

Downey G, Coyne JC: Children of depressed parents: an integrative review. Psychol Bull 108(1):50–76, 1990 2200073

Elliot RL, Campbell L, Hunter M, et al: When I look into my baby's eyes…infant emotion recognition by mothers with borderline personality disorder. Infant Ment Health J 35(1):21–32, 2014 25424403

Eve PM, Byrne MK, Gagliardi CR: What is good parenting? The perspectives of different professionals. Family Court Review 52(1):114–127, 2014

Famularo R, Kinscherff R, Fenton T: Psychiatric diagnoses of abusive mothers. A preliminary report. J Nerv Ment Dis 180(10):658–661, 1992 1402845

Fonagy P: Affect Regulation, Mentalization and the Development of the Self. New York, Other Press, 2002

Forrester D: Parental substance misuse and child protection in a British sample. A survey of children on the Child Protection Register in an inner London district office. Child Abuse Review 9(4):235–246, 2000

Frick PJ, Lahey BB, Loeber R, et al: Familial risk factors to oppositional defiant disorder and conduct disorder: parental psychopathology and maternal parenting. J Consult Clin Psychol 60(1):49–55, 1992 1556285

Gabbard GO: Psychodynamic Psychiatry in Clinical Practice. Washington, DC, American Psychiatric Publishing, 2014

Grant BF, Hasin DS, Stinson FS, et al: Prevalence, correlates, and disability of personality disorders in the United States: results from the National Epidemiologic Survey on Alcohol and Related Conditions. J Clin Psychiatry 65(7):948–958, 2004 15291684

Haarer J: Die Deutsche Mutter und ihr Erstes Kind. Munich, Lehmann, 1943

Herr NR, Hammen C, Brennan PA: Maternal borderline personality disorder symptoms and adolescent psychosocial functioning. J Pers Disord 22(5):451–465, 2008 18834294

Hobson RP, Patrick M, Crandell L, et al: Personal relatedness and attachment in infants of mothers with borderline personality disorder. Dev Psychopathol 17(2):329–347, 2005 16761548

Holtzworth-Munroe A: A typology of men who are violent toward their female partners: making sense of the heterogeneity in husband violence. Current Directions in Psychological Science 9(4):140–143, 2000

Johnson JG, Cohen P, Smailes EM, et al: Childhood verbal abuse and risk for personality disorders during adolescence and early adulthood. Compr Psychiatry 42(1):16–23, 2001 11154711

Johnson JG, Cohen P, Kasen S, et al: Associations of parental personality disorders and Axis I disorders with childrearing behavior. Psychiatry 69(4):336–350, 2006 17326728

Johnson JG, Cohen P, Kasen S, et al: Psychiatric disorders in adolescence and early adulthood and risk for child-rearing difficulties during middle adulthood. Journal of Family Issues 29(2):210–233, 2008

Kaess M, von Ceumern-Lindenstjerna I-A, Parzer P, et al: Axis I and II comorbidity and psychosocial functioning in female adolescents with borderline personality disorder. Psychopathology 46(1):55–62, 2013 22890504

Kellett J, Apps J: Assessments of parenting and parenting support need: a study of four professional groups. Joseph Roundtree Foundation, August 2009. Available at: https://www.jrf.org.uk/sites/default/files/jrf/migrated/files/parenting-support-need-full.pdf. Accessed April 16, 2019.

Kendler KS: Parenting: a genetic-epidemiologic perspective. Am J Psychiatry 153(1):11–20, 1996 8540566

Lahey BB, Piacentini JC, McBurnett K, et al: Psychopathology in the parents of children with conduct disorder and hyperactivity. J Am Acad Child Adolesc Psychiatry 27(2):163–170, 1988 3360717

Laulik S, Chou S, Browne KD, et al: The link between personality disorder and parenting behaviors: a systematic review. Aggression and Violent Behavior 18:644–655, 2013

Lees J, Manning N, Rawlings B: Therapeutic Community Effectiveness: A Systematic International Review of Therapeutic Community Treatment for People With Personality Disorders and Mentally Disordered Offenders. York, UK, NHS Centre for Reviews and Dissemination, 1999

Lenzenweger MF, Lane MC, Loranger AW, et al: DSM-IV personality disorders in the National Comorbidity Survey Replication. Biol Psychiatry 62(6):553–564, 2007 17217923

Levy KN, Meehan KB, Weber M, et al: Attachment and borderline personality disorder: implications for psychotherapy. Psychopathology 38(2):64–74, 2005 15802944

Levy KN, McMain S, Bateman A, et al: Treatment of borderline personality disorder. Psychiatr Clin North Am 41(4):711–728, 2018 30447734

Lydecker JA, Grilo CM: Fathers and mothers with eating-disorder psychopathology: associations with child eating-disorder behaviors. J Psychosom Res 86:63–69, 2016 27302549

McGlashan TH, Grilo CM, Skodol AE, et al: The Collaborative Longitudinal Personality Disorders Study: baseline Axis I/II and II/II diagnostic co-occurrence. Acta Psychiatr Scand 102(4):256–264, 2000 11089725

McMurran M, Huband N, Overton E: Non-completion of personality disorder treatments: a systematic review of correlates, consequences, and interventions. Clin Psychol Rev 30(3):277–287, 2010 20047783

Meyer B, Pilkonis PA, Beevers CG: What's in a (neutral) face? Personality disorders, attachment styles, and the appraisal of ambiguous social cues. J Pers Disord 18(4):320–336, 2004 15342321

Newman L, Stevenson C: Parenting and borderline personality disorder: ghosts in the nursery. Clin Child Psychol Psychiatry 10(3):385–394, 2005

Newman LK, Stevenson CS, Bergman LR, et al: Borderline personality disorder, mother-infant interaction and parenting perceptions: preliminary findings. Aust NZ J Psychiatry 41(7):598–605, 2007 17558622

Nickell AD, Waudby CJ, Trull TJ: Attachment, parental bonding and borderline personality disorder features in young adults. J Pers Disord 16(2):148–159, 2002 12004491

Niesten IJ, Karan E, Frankenburg FR, et al: Description and prediction of the income status of borderline patients over 10 years of prospective follow-up. Pers Ment Health 10(4):285–292, 2016 26864557

Nigg JT, Hinshaw SP: Parent personality traits and psychopathology associated with antisocial behaviors in childhood attention-deficit hyperactivity disorder. J Child Psychol Psychiatry 39(2):145–159, 1998 9669228

Nordahl HM, Stiles TC: Perceptions of parental bonding in patients with various personality disorders, lifetime depressive disorders, and healthy controls. J Pers Disord 11(4):391–402, 1997 9484698

Paris J, Zweig-Frank H, Guzder J: Psychological risk factors for borderline personality disorder in female patients. Compr Psychiatry 35(4):301–305, 1994 7956187

Perry JC, Bond M, Roy C: Predictors of treatment duration and retention in a study of long-term dynamic psychotherapy: childhood adversity, adult personality, and diagnosis. J Psychiatr Pract 13(4):221–232, 2007 17667734

Petfield L, Startup H, Droscher H, et al: Parenting in mothers with borderline personality disorder and impact on child outcomes. Evid Based Ment Health 18(3):67–75, 2015 26205740

Royal College of Psychiatrists: Parents as patients: supporting the needs of patients who are parents and their children. College Report CR164, January 2011. Available at: https://www.rcpsych.ac.uk/docs/default-source/members/faculties/perinatal-psychiatry/perinatal-reports-cr164.pdf?sfvrsn=1ed25435_2. Accessed April 16, 2019.

Samuels J, Bienvenu OJ 3rd, Riddle MA, et al: Hoarding in obsessive compulsive disorder: results from a case-control study. Behav Res Ther 40(5):517–528, 2002 12043707

Schacht R, Hammond L, Marks M, et al: The relation between mind-mindedness in mothers with borderline personality disorder and mental state understanding in their children. Infant and Child Development 22(1):68–84, 2013

Shea MT, Widiger TA, Klein MH: Comorbidity of personality disorders and depression: implications for treatment. J Consult Clin Psychol 60(6):857–868, 1992 1460149

South SC, Turkheimer E, Oltmanns TF: Personality disorder symptoms and marital functioning. J Consult Clin Psychol 76(5):769–780, 2008 18837594

Sperry L: Handbook of Diagnosis and Treatment of DSM-IV-TR Personality Disorders, 2nd Edition. New York, Brunner-Routledge, 2003

Sperry L: Cognitive Behavior Therapy of DSM-IV-TR Personality Disorders: Highly Effective Interventions for the Most Common Personality Disorders, 2nd Edition. New York, Routledge, 2006

Torgersen S, Kringlen E, Cramer V: The prevalence of personality disorders in a community sample. Arch Gen Psychiatry 58(6):590–596, 2001 11386989

Verhage ML, Schuengel C, Madigan S, et al: Narrowing the transmission gap: a synthesis of three decades of research on intergenerational transmission of attachment. Psychol Bull 142(4):337–366, 2016 26653864

Westen D, Harnden-Fischer J: Personality profiles in eating disorders: rethinking the distinction between Axis I and Axis II. Am J Psychiatry 158(4):547–562, 2001 11282688

White RJ, Gondolf EW: Implications of personality profiles for batterer treatment. Journal of Interpersonal Violence 15(5):467–488, 2000

Wiehe VR: Empathy and narcissism in a sample of child abuse perpetrators and a comparison sample of foster parents. Child Abuse Negl 27(5):541–555, 2003 12718962

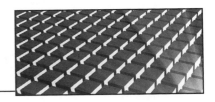

CHAPTER 12

POSITIVE ASPECTS
OF OCPD

Samuel R. Chamberlain, M.B./B.Chir., Ph.D., M.R.C.Psych.
Jon E. Grant, M.D., M.P.H., J.D.

Case Vignette

Mavis is a 33-year-old senior administrator in a hospital clinic. She is a stickler for the rules, tends to shun close social contact (stating that "the workplace is for work, not fun"), and insists on high standards. When staff submit expense claim forms, Mavis is careful to check that they are accurate and complete, and she rejects them even for minor rule breaches. Mavis keeps the staff kitchen highly organized and has a vigilant eye—for example, she scolds people for using the milk without making the appropriate contribution to the staff tea and coffee fund. She works longer hours than anyone else but does not request overtime pay (knowing that the company does not have funds for overtime). Mavis knows how to get things done and has extensive knowledge of the rules regarding the hospital and administrative matters. She is contented with her approach to life and does not mind not having close friends or interests outside of her job. Opinion among other staff is mixed: some people appreciate Mavis's dedication to work and efficiency, whereas others find her frustrating because their expense claims are rejected often. Mavis's boss is extremely pleased with her because the department passed a recent financial audit with 100% scores; however, a staff member has filed a complaint about Mavis because she was rude and dismissive to him.

Although obsessive-compulsive personality disorder (OCPD) is by definition functionally impairing (American Psychiatric Association 2013), it is important to question whether having some traits of OCPD could in fact be functionally useful or adaptive. If so, this may help to account for why OCPD traits persist over time in humans. As explored elsewhere in this book, OCPD is characterized at its core by rigidity and inflexibility at the expense of efficiency and interpersonal interactions, occurring in multiple situations and beginning by early adulthood. Additionally, four or more of the following concrete criteria need to be met for the diagnosis: preoccupation with rules, perfectionism interfering with task completion, overdevotion to work and productivity, an inflexible values system, hoarding, reluctance to delegate, strictness with money, and rigidity and stubbornness. Intuitively, if one removes the functional impairment elements of these criteria, one would be left with a set of personality traits that could in fact be helpful or useful in some occupations or social settings. Also, conceivably, even if someone has a diagnosis of OCPD, there could be situations in which those symptoms are adaptive or positive, even if they are viewed as generally impairing in most settings.

POSITIVE SOCIAL AND COGNITIVE ASSOCIATIONS WITH OCPD

Because OCPD is conceptualized as a pathology, there is little research into whether OCPD itself—at the full level or trait level—could be functionally useful or adaptive. In a rare exception to this lack of research, Ullrich et al. (2007) studied dimensions of personality disorder and life success in a sample of 304 middle-age men recruited from the general community. They found that the OCPD dimension was positively correlated with status and wealth; notably, this was the only positive relationship with status and wealth that would have retained statistical significance with Bonferroni correction. Other dimensions of personality disorder (schizoid, schizotypal, antisocial) had negative associations with status and wealth. In terms of successful intimate relationships, the OCPD dimension did not have a statistically significant association, whereas negative associations were found for avoidant, dependent, schizotypal, schizoid, borderline, and antisocial personality disorder dimensions. This study indicates that dimensional aspects of OCPD can have positive associations, but interpretation is tempered by the many negative associations reported in the literature for OCPD itself.

One vantage point for understanding possible negative and positive associations with OCPD is cognitive research. Logically, the core symptoms of OCPD suggest rigid response styles, meaning that a person may try to find the perfect solution even if doing so interferes with task completion. Alternatively, it could be reasoned that perfectionist traits could be useful on some cognitive tasks because the individual might work harder to seek out optimal solutions than would someone without OCPD.

Is there any evidence to support the idea that some cognitive functions may be superior in people with OCPD compared with control subjects? In a study that compared people with comorbid OCPD and OCD with people with only OCD, those with comorbidity had significantly worse set shifting (difficulty inhibiting and shifting attention away from a previously relevant stimulus dimension onto a different previously irrelevant stimulus dimension) (Fineberg et al. 2007). This is in keeping with the linking of OCPD with cognitive rigidity. Set-shifting deficits, along with executive planning deficits, have also been found in nonclinical cases of OCPD compared with control subjects (Fineberg et al. 2015). Set-shifting and executive planning tasks are dependent on the functioning of the dorsolateral prefrontal cortices, raising the possibility that these regions may play a role in OCPD. These cognitive results indicate deficits rather than better functioning in OCPD, consistent with a pathological tendency to stick with what was previously correct or with what the individual believes *should be* correct according to his or her own rules. Although direct evidence is lacking, these tendencies could be adaptive if manifested to a lesser degree, as may be anticipated in people with OCPD traits rather than the full disorder.

In another cognitive study, monetary discounting was examined in four groups: individuals with OCPD, those with OCD, those with both disorders, and healthy control subjects (Pinto et al. 2014). *Discounting* refers to a preference for more immediate short-term rewards over larger but delayed rewards. Discounting is typically elevated in impulsive individuals, such as those with substance use disorders, attention-deficit hyperactivity disorder (ADHD), or antisocial personality disorder (e.g., Jackson and MacKillop 2016). The group with "pure" OCPD had a higher capacity to defer or delay reward compared with the comorbid OCPD+OCD group and a control group; the OCD group did not differ from the control group (Pinto et al. 2014). Because discounting is typically interpreted as a deficit (as in ADHD and other disorders listed above), the capacity to delay reward could be viewed as a relative cognitive benefit in OCPD; however, it is not known whether this less steep discounting function in OCPD is functionally useful.

BROADER MEASUREMENT OF PERSONALITY TRAITS: INSIGHTS INTO OCPD

Because of a lack of data regarding possible positive aspects of OCPD, we must turn to studies of personality measures in other frameworks, especially the five-factor model (FFM; McCrae and John 1992). The FFM was originally developed on the basis of findings from natural language studies as a means of understanding the normal range of personalities (i.e., how we describe people) and other frameworks. The FFM typically includes five personality domains: openness to experience, conscientiousness, extroversion, agreeableness, and neuroticism. Several meta-analyses of the available literature have shown that OCPD is associated with higher levels of conscientiousness, measured using the NEO Personality Inventory—Revised (NEO-PI-R), whereas the other personality domains have been shown to be relatively unrelated to OCPD (Samuel and Widiger 2008; Saulsman and Page 2004). When the questions on the NEO-PI-R used to assess conscientiousness were modified to reflect impairment (e.g., adding terms such as "excessively" or "preoccupied"), the association between conscientiousness and OCPD was more pronounced (Haigler and Widiger 2001). Similar findings linking OCPD to high levels of conscientiousness have also been documented with other psychological instruments, including the Temperament and Character Inventory (TCI; Samuel and Gore 2012), suggesting that this is a replicable, true association.

CONSCIENTIOUSNESS AND COGNITION

Some studies have explored whether conscientiousness may relate to cognition. Conceivably, conscientiousness could incorporate a strong preference for making correct decisions or avoiding errors, which could be helpful on some cognitive tasks. In individuals with traumatic brain injuries, damage to the dorsolateral prefrontal cortices was associated with low conscientiousness and with lower scores on executive function tests plus measures of psychomotor speed (Forbes et al. 2014), and it is tempting to speculate the corollary—that high conscientiousness may be linked with superior cognitive function. In a 7-year study in older people, higher conscientiousness was linked with slower age-related cognitive decline (as indexed by total scores on the Mini-Mental State Examination), even after controlling for many potential confounding variables (Chapman et al. 2012). Unfortunately, there is a relative poverty of research into whether conscientiousness is associated with better performance in discrete cognitive domains rather than more global measures.

POSITIVE ASSOCIATIONS WITH CONSCIENTIOUSNESS IN YOUTH THROUGH TO MIDDLE AGE

Conscientiousness and other personality traits have been fairly widely studied in relation to academic and occupational functioning and occupational success. This is perhaps not surprising because traits of high standards and perfectionism may be especially valued in such contexts. In a study of 300 adolescent boys, inverse factor analysis was used to identify separable personality types based on the California Child Q-Set (CCQ), which asks caregivers to indicate personality descriptions for a given child on the basis of 100 items printed on individual cards (sorted into nine categories from extremely uncharacteristic to extremely characteristic) (Robins et al. 1996). This sorting yielded three types: a personally and socially well-adjusted group (group 1); an inhibited, somewhat anxious, but otherwise socially agreeable group (group 2); and an antisocial group (group 3). The structure of these groups was confirmed across different ethnic groupings. Conscientiousness scores were high for group 1, moderate for group 2, and low for group 3.

Blatný et al. (2015) conducted a longitudinal study that was first initiated in the 1960s with toddlers; follow-up data were collected when participants were age 16 years and again in 2001 (during adulthood) where feasible. In the adult data set analyzed cross-sectionally, personality traits including conscientiousness were significantly correlated with higher self-esteem, life satisfaction, and self-efficacy. This result supports the notion that the conscientiousness component of OCPD traits has positive rather than negative functional connotations. Conscientiousness was not measured in the earlier elements of the study (childhood and teenager years).

Could conscientiousness be particularly related to elements of scholarly or vocational performance success in students? Rhee and colleagues (2013) explored how personality related to aspects of teamwork in university students. Student teams were largely self-selected (e.g., a group tending to work together within a particular subject class), and five-factor personality scores were recorded. The results indicated that conscientiousness was significantly correlated with an individual's self-reported scores for engagement in discussions, taking a leadership role, contributing useful ideas, encouraging the group to complete tasks on time, and clear communication. Conscientiousness had more significant positive correlations with aspects of team working than did the other big five personality traits that were examined. In a study of medical residents, higher levels of conscientiousness reported by the students were significantly associated with higher professionalism ratings as judged by their faculty supervisors (Phillips et al. 2018). Faculty members rated conscientiousness as the second most important personality trait for residents, whereas residents rated conscientiousness as the fifth most important personality trait. If this finding generalizes, it may indicate that people may perceive conscientiousness as being important in others but less so in themselves.

Moes and colleagues (1996) studied personality traits of 100 successful Navy submarine staff, all at the rank of chief petty officer or above. The Schedule for Non-Adaptive and Adaptive Personality (SNAP) was used. The mean personality trait scale scores for the whole group were fairly typical compared with external normative data, although matched control data were not available. The trait scores most descriptive of the sample were workaholism, detachment, and propriety—namely, those that would be expected to be related to OCPD tendencies. Thirty-seven percent of the sample had diagnostic scale scores indicative of probable personality disorder. The most common likely personality disorders were antisocial (15%), obsessive-compulsive (9%), and avoidant (8%) types. The high rate of antisocial personality is interesting because this result would fit with the idea that some people with antisocial tendencies may adapt well to military life, perhaps because of rigid boundaries and opportunities for progression. The link with OCPD is in keeping with the view that these traits are not necessarily a barrier to success in particular career settings and, in fact, may in some ways be adaptive, even though they are typically regarded as diagnostically negative and impairing.

Some studies have explored how personality traits, including conscientiousness, relate to income. In general, higher levels of conscientiousness have been shown to be associated with higher income levels across multiple research studies (for detailed discussion, see Denissen et al. 2018). In a large German study of employed people ($N=8,458$), the relationships between actual and job-required personality traits and income were characterized (Denissen et al. 2018). Interestingly, job demands of conscientiousness were typically higher than actual levels of these traits among the workforce, suggesting that there were not enough conscientious people to satisfy the local labor market requirements. In contrast, for traits of extroversion, agreeableness, and openness to experience, the expression and job requirements were relatively well matched. Intriguingly, people with high conscientiousness in jobs with low demands for this trait had lower rather than higher income. Thus, it would appear that the OCPD trait of conscientiousness is associated with greater income but only when this trait is important to the job. Conceivably, highly conscientious people in mismatched roles could be penalized and be less successful than peers.

POSITIVE ASSOCIATIONS WITH CONSCIENTIOUSNESS IN OLDER AGE GROUPS

Baek et al. (2016) examined whether personality traits in older adults (age 80 years and older) were related to different aspects of successful aging. The authors extracted two higher-order factor scores for the personality traits: alpha (conscientiousness, agreeableness, and neuroticism) and beta (extroversion and openness to experience). This two-factor model has also been used in other areas of personality research and derives from Digman's (1997) research in this area. Baek and colleagues conducted regression modeling, controlling for such variables as age, gender, and ethnicity. Higher alpha scores were associated with better cognition, more volunteering, more activities of daily living, and higher levels of subjective health.

CONSCIENTIOUSNESS AND RESILIENCE: POTENTIAL IMPLICATIONS FOR OCPD

In all, conscientiousness is likely to be an important determinant of some areas of functioning across the lifespan. Why might conscientiousness have such positive longitudinal associations across the lifespan? One possibility is that conscientiousness confers resilience. Resilience refers to the ability of a person to be successful (or to function well) despite stressful or untoward circumstances (van Harmelen et al. 2017). For example, an individual with an extremely difficult, socially and economically deprived childhood who then goes on to become high functioning in adulthood would be said to be highly resilient. In a sample of 130 undergraduate students in Japan (Nakaya et al. 2006), moderate positive correlations were found between conscientiousness and higher adolescent resilience. Indeed, this correlation had the largest positive effect size versus the other big five personality traits, although neuroticism had a larger effect in the opposite direction—in other words, high conscientiousness and low neuroticism were associated with higher resilience (Nakaya et al. 2006). Also in support of this hypothesis, in 693 male participants in the Terman Life Cycle Study, conscientiousness predicted lower mortality, especially in relatively unsuccessful individuals (Figure 12–1) (Kern et al. 2009).

CONCLUSION

Very few studies have sought to characterize OCPD as having any positive or beneficial associations, given that the disorder is defined by the fundamental assumption of persistent, marked functional impairment. Apart from one study suggesting that OCPD traits were linked with higher status and wealth (Ullrich et al. 2007), the majority of studies have focused on categorical OCPD and reported negative associations, as considered in chapters throughout this book. Nonetheless, a focus on dimensional personality domains germane to OCPD has yielded interesting insights. Conscientiousness has been associated with better functioning in some domains, including academic and work outcomes, ability to work on a team, slower age-related cognitive decline, and lower mortality (for the latter, especially in less successful people, see Figure 12–1). One explanation proffered here that may account for these lifespan associations is that conscientiousness may confer resilience. There is also initial evidence that categorical OCPD may be associated with a heightened ability to defer gratification (Pinto et al. 2014), although it is not known whether this ability is adaptive or useful, and other important cognitive domains have been shown to be markedly impaired in individuals with OCPD (Fineberg et al. 2007, 2015). Further research into OCPD traits, fractionated into latent factors (rather than considering OCPD as a unitary phenomenon), is needed to explore potentially adaptive elements of OCPD.

CASE VIGNETTE DISCUSSION

In the case vignette, Mavis exhibits features that would meet criteria for OCPD; however, she feels that her personality is a positive thing and that it is not associated with functional impairment. This raises the interesting issue of who judges whether a set of personality traits constitutes a disorder or not: a clinician may identify perceived functional impairment by using his or her own set of standards and expectations, which may or may not match those of society. An interesting thought experiment would be to imagine what Mavis's coworkers would think if asked whether her personality is useful or problematic. Presumably some would view her tendencies as positive ("She is a highly efficient

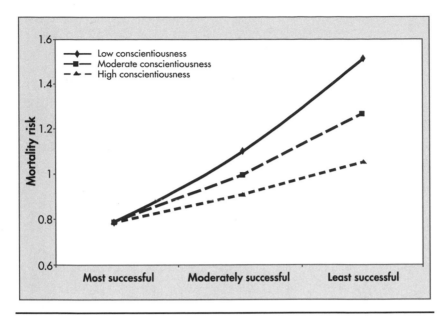

FIGURE 12–1. Conscientiousness and career success.

Lifespan data show that conscientiousness is associated with lower mortality risk per time frame, especially in less successful individuals.

Source. Reprinted from Kern ML, Friedman HS, Martin LR, et al.: "Conscientiousness, Career Success, and Longevity: A Lifespan Analysis." *Annals of Behavioral Medicine* 37(2):154–163, 2009. Copyright © 2009 Oxford University Press. Used with permission.

worker"), whereas others would view her approach as negative ("She is too strict," "She upsets people by her directness," "She stops me from achieving my goals at work because she applies rules too firmly"). There is also the issue of situational importance: if these traits are desirable in some types of employment but problematic in others, do they, in fact, constitute a disorder? The case vignette raises a number of questions that unfortunately cannot be answered and instead highlight a lack of research into whether trait features of OCPD are useful. The most research relevant to this is work on conscientiousness, which has a number of reported positive lifespan associations.

TAKE-HOME POINTS

- Sustained functional impairment is central to the definition of OCPD; hence, the overwhelming majority of research into OCPD has focused on negative rather than potentially positive associations.

- Conscientiousness is associated with OCPD, and research links conscientiousness to better scholastic and occupational functioning across the lifespan and even to lower mortality rates. This apparent paradox (OCPD being impairing, but conscientiousness having positive associations) could be related to the extent to which a trait is manifested. For example, moderate conscientiousness may be useful, whereas extreme conscientiousness becomes pathological. Additionally, other elements of personality may also be important in determining the impact of OCPD traits.

- We hypothesize that moderate conscientiousness may confer resilience, which, in turn, may account for some of its positive long-term associations across the age span.

- In order to understand aspects of OCPD that have positive associations, future work should use a dimensional approach, examining latent forms of OCPD, ideally incorporating measurement indices that are neutrally worded (rather than worded only with a negative emphasis).

REFERENCES

American Psychiatric Association: Diagnostic and Statistical Manual of Mental Disorders, 5th Edition. Arlington, VA, American Psychiatric Association, 2013

Baek Y, Martin P, Siegler IC, et al: Personality traits and successful aging: findings from the Georgia Centenarian Study. Int J Aging Hum Dev 83(3):207–227, 2016 27298487

Blatný M, Millová K, Jelínek M, et al: Personality predictors of successful development: toddler temperament and adolescent personality traits predict well-being and career stability in middle adulthood. PLoS One 10(4):e0126032, 2015 25919394

Chapman B, Duberstein P, Tindle HA, et al; Gingko Evaluation of Memory Study Investigators: Personality predicts cognitive function over 7 years in older persons. Am J Geriatr Psychiatry 20(7):612–621, 2012 22735597

Denissen JJA, Bleidorn W, Hennecke M, et al: Uncovering the power of personality to shape income. Psychol Sci 29(1):3–13, 2018 29155616

Digman JM: Higher-order factors of the big five. J Pers Soc Psychol 73(6):1246–1256, 1997 9418278

Fineberg NA, Sharma P, Sivakumaran T, et al: Does obsessive-compulsive personality disorder belong within the obsessive-compulsive spectrum? CNS Spectr 12(6):467–482, 2007 17545957

Fineberg NA, Day GA, de Koenigswarter N, et al: The neuropsychology of obsessive-compulsive personality disorder: a new analysis. CNS Spectr 20(5):490–499, 2015 25776273

Forbes CE, Poore JC, Krueger F, et al: The role of executive function and the dorsolateral prefrontal cortex in the expression of neuroticism and conscientiousness. Soc Neurosci 9(2):139–151, 2014 24405294

Haigler ED, Widiger TA: Experimental manipulation of NEO-PI-R items. J Pers Assess 77(2):339–358, 2001 11693863

Jackson JN, MacKillop J: Attention-deficit/hyperactivity disorder and monetary delay discounting: a meta-analysis of case-control studies. Biol Psychiatry Cogn Neurosci Neuroimaging 1(4):316–325, 2016 27722208

Kern ML, Friedman HS, Martin LR, et al: Conscientiousness, career success, and longevity: a lifespan analysis. Ann Behav Med 37(2):154–163, 2009 19455378

McCrae RR, John OP: An introduction to the five-factor model and its applications. J Pers 60(2):175–215, 1992 1635039

Moes GS, Lall R, Johnson WB: Personality characteristics of successful Navy submarine personnel. Mil Med 161(4):239–242, 1996 8935516

Nakaya M, Oshio A, Kaneko H: Correlations for Adolescent Resilience Scale with big five personality traits. Psychol Rep 98(3):927–930, 2006 16933700

Phillips D, Egol KA, Maculatis MC, et al: Personality factors associated with resident performance: results from 12 Accreditation Council for Graduate Medical Education accredited orthopaedic surgery programs. J Surg Educ 75(1):122–131, 2018 28688967

Pinto A, Steinglass JE, Greene AL, et al: Capacity to delay reward differentiates obsessive-compulsive disorder and obsessive-compulsive personality disorder. Biol Psychiatry 75(8):653–659, 2014 24199665

Rhee J, Parent D, Basu A: The influence of personality and ability on undergraduate teamwork and team performance. Springerplus 2(1):16, 2013 23420685

Robins RW, John OP, Caspi A, et al: Resilient, overcontrolled, and undercontrolled boys: three replicable personality types. J Pers Soc Psychol 70(1):157–171, 1996 8558407

Samuel DB, Gore WL: Maladaptive variants of conscientiousness and agreeableness. J Pers 80(6):1669–1696, 2012 22321159

Samuel DB, Widiger TA: A meta-analytic review of the relationships between the five-factor model and DSM-IV-TR personality disorders: a facet level analysis. Clin Psychol Rev 28(8):1326–1342, 2008 18708274

Saulsman LM, Page AC: The five-factor model and personality disorder empirical literature: a meta-analytic review. Clin Psychol Rev 23(8):1055–1085, 2004 14729423

Ullrich S, Farrington DP, Coid JW: Dimensions of DSM-IV personality disorders and life-success. J Pers Disord 21(6):657–663, 2007 18072866

van Harmelen AL, Kievit RA, Ioannidis K, et al: Adolescent friendships predict later resilient functioning across psychosocial domains in a healthy community cohort. Psychol Med 47(13):2312–2322, 2017 28397612

INDEX

Page numbers printed in **boldface** type refer to tables and figures.